What Healthy People Know

And the 7 things they do to stay healthy and live long

Dr. Bob Gleeson, M.D.

Health Now, LLC

in association with

Classic Day Publishing

Seattle, Washington
Portland, Oregon
Denver, Colorado
Vancouver, B.C.
Scottsdale, Arizona
Minneapolis, Minnesota

Health Now, LLC
in association with
Classic Day Publishing
2207 Fairview Avenue East, #4
Seattle, Washington 98102
www.classicdaypublishing.com

FOREWORD

As a United States Senator, I believe we need to fundamentally reorient our approach to health care in America toward disease prevention and wellness. I have introduced the Healthy Lifestyles and Prevention Act (HeLP America Act), federal legislation to promote good health. The aim is to give individuals and communities the information and tools they need to take charge of their own health. Dr. Bob Gleeson's book, *What Healthy People Know,* gives us that information. His book tells us exactly how much difference a healthy lifestyle makes. He gives us the supporting science and tells us how we can each live a disease-free life. The science and his guidance are very clear and compelling.

In the United States, we fail to make an up-front investment in prevention. So we end up spending hundreds of billions on hospitalization, treatment, and disability. This is foolish—and, clearly, unsustainable. In fact, I've long said that we don't have a health care system here in America, we have a "sick care" system. And it is costing us dearly, both in terms of health care costs and premature deaths.

I don't think you'll find too many people who would argue with the statement that if you get sick, the best place in the world to get the care you need is here in America. We have the best trained, highest-skilled health professionals in the world. We have cutting-edge, state-of-the-art equipment and technology. We have world-class health care facilities and research institutions.

But when it comes to helping people stay healthy and out of the hospital, we fall woefully short. In the U.S., we spend in excess of $1.8 trillion a year on health care. Fully 75 percent of that total is accounted for by chronic diseases—things like heart disease, cancer, and diabetes. And many of these diseases are largely preventable.

Now, if I bought a new car, drove that car off the lot, and never maintained it—never checked the oil, never checked the transmission fluid, never got it tuned up—you'd think I was crazy, not to mention grossly irresponsible. The common-sense principle with an automobile is: "I pay a little now to keep the car maintained, or I pay a whole lot later."

Well, it's the same with our national health priorities. Right now, our health care system is in a downward spiral. We are not paying a little now, so we are paying a whole lot later. If we are serious about getting control of health care costs and health insurance premiums, we must give people access to information so they can make good decisions about their own health.

It's time to read and follow the clear and scientifically supported advice in this book. If everyone started to follow these simple prescriptions, we could substantially reduce chronic disease and promote health. And that would be good for all Americans.

— Tom Harkin, United States Senator

This book is dedicated to my parents,
Helen Jane and Robert E.

Their loving, generous, and active lives
are an inspiration to me.

ACKNOWLEDGMENTS

Although written by one person, every book represents a group adventure. Every author needs the encouragement and support of family and friends. I thank everyone who encouraged me, questioned me, prodded me, and helped me.

I wish to thank the professionals who stood in my corner through thick and thin:

- ◆ Elliott Wolf of Classic Day Publishing, because he believed in me when other agents and publishers did not.

- ◆ Anne Greenberg, my New York editor, who saw the nugget among the dross I first sent her. And then did the final polishing.

- ◆ Jude Neuman, word doctor par excellence, who taught this science doctor how to write a clear sentence.

- ◆ Amy Vaughn and David Marty of David Marty Design, who made the manuscript, graphs, and tables clearly tell a consistent story.

- ◆ Sharon Memory, MPH, who made certain that all of the myriad of facts, even the spelling of my own name, were correct.

- ◆ Dan Drummond, who did the final proofreading while maintaining my language and tone.

- ◆ Ken Swoyer of Cobey Communications, who knows how to capture the essence of a book into a headline.

- ◆ Rick Frishman of Planned Television Arts, for his enthusiastic support and admission to his wonderful network.

- ◆ Eric Kampmann and Gail Krump of Midpoint Trade Books, who know "a thing or two about books."

I wish to thank all of my friends who listened to my endless stories. Their support never wavered, and they provided me with a deep understanding of the fine nature of their personal character. This includes Ken and Louise, Pam and Marty, Bruce and Janine, and Bill and Barb.

I must sincerely thank all of my friends at Northwestern Mutual, the finest financial security company in America. Their individual and personal encouragement sustained me as I wrote in predawn hours.

I wish to thank my family. My wonderful bride of 30 years, Jane, is always loving, supportive, and intellectually way ahead of me; she is largely responsible for all of the successful details that make this book work. My three children, Elizabeth, Megan, and Rob, always believed in my ability to do this. They helped in editing and reading. Don't worry, kids, I am almost done with this book and can soon return to cooking dinner again.

PATIENT TESTIMONIALS

"I had to have a heart attack before I could hear Dr. Bob's message of why good health mattered and how to get there. I suggest you read this book before you have your own heart attack. As Dr. Bob says, 'It is far better to prevent a heart attack than to treat it well.'"

— R W

"Dr. Bob gave me back my life. Three years ago I was significantly overweight, out of shape, and had lost belief that I could recapture my health. Dr. Bob's encouragement and discussions on a sustainable program of healthy eating and exercise helped me to change the pattern of my life and allowed me to recapture control of my own life. He showed and encouraged me to lose over 150 pounds and keep it off for more than 3 years. I am strong again, eat well, and feel good about myself. I did nothing other than follow Dr. Bob's prescriptions inside this book. Regaining my health was not complicated, difficult, or unpleasant. My good health has been a simple and wonderful gift."

— S K

"A few years ago, Dr. Bob gave me a prescription to improve my health. He told me to go for a walk and eat an apple every day. A year later I have lost over 50 pounds and regained a very large measure of both self-respect and strength. I love the new me. Thank you, Dr. Bob."

— F C

CONTENTS

"Middle-aged adults in low-risk groups have an 80% lower rate of death from coronary heart disease than adults in average-risk groups. That's an astounding difference. Unfortunately, only a small percentage of adults are at low risk. Our challenge for the 21st century is to prevent risk factors from developing in the first place by encouraging healthy behaviors early in life."

— *Dr. Claude Lenfant*
Former Director of the National Heart Lung and Blood Institute of the National Institutes of Health (with permission)

PREFACE

Better health with less disease. Living a longer life—maybe even to 90—with vigor. Wishful thinking? Science fiction? Ambitions for the next millennium? No.

Such goals are attainable in the here and now. And you may be surprised to learn that everyone can achieve these goals. It's happening already. People who consistently make healthy choices have astonishingly long and active lives. Their risk of chronic disease is very low, and they can expect to live to a very active old age, with few medical problems. These people have been studied, and the research confirms it: we are at a point in history where, if we take care of ourselves, we can expect to avoid the diseases typically linked to aging—and live active, long lives.

Yet the fact of the matter is that many of us are slightly (or more than slightly) overweight and out of shape. We know we should do something about it, but we're not sure what to do. Several times a week, the news bombards us with conflicting messages about how to eat right, weigh less, and exercise more.

Confused and overwhelmed, we do nothing. Yet there is a path to better health. What's more, this path is neither complicated nor difficult.

On the path are the health choices we face every day, all day long. To achieve better health, we just have to make an informed choice: avoid the unhealthy and choose the healthy. This book will help you do that—and no choice is much more complex than figuring out when to eat "an apple a day."

I promise you, these small, daily choices do matter tremendously. Cumulatively, they make substantial short- and long-term differences in your health: how often you get sick, how quickly you get well, the cost of your health care—and ultimately, how long you live.

HOW DO I KNOW?

For the past 25 years, I have worked as the medical director of a major life insurance company. Part of my job has been determining how long I thought you might live. In the process, I have discovered that the healthiest people are sick less often, spend fewer health care dollars, and live longer than those with average health—and far longer than those with poor health habits. The numbers make a strong case for actively pursuing better health.

As I continue to learn more about the health habits and choices of the healthiest people, I become more and more convinced that everyone could and would become healthier if only they understood how simple and how close to good health they already are. I've been amazed at how quickly a person can move from unhealthy to healthy. Once I understood the cumulative effect of these differences, I quietly changed my own daily health choices. I would like to help you change yours.

WHY I CARE

Preventive medicine has always fascinated me. In medical school, I wanted to specialize in this field, but at the time, 1974, the federal government reduced funds for preventive medicine residencies. So I specialized in internal medicine instead. I treated sick patients for a few years, but I was constantly reminded of how an ounce of prevention was worth a pound of cure.

In the early 1980s, I found myself applying to the Mayo Clinic and Harvard for further study in preventive medicine. However, you know how these things go: start down one path, and suddenly you find yourself somewhere else in life. Me, too. On my way to a high-powered preventive medicine program, I took a turn in the road. I was lucky enough to be hired as a full-time medical director for a well-respected and prominent life insurance company.

My position enabled me to practice what I call "applied preventive medicine." As medical director, I studied the medical risks and life expectancies of life insurance applicants. What level of blood pressure or cholesterol was low enough for the longest life? How much weight was too much? What were the differences between unhealthy and healthy people?

WHAT I LEARNED IN THE WORLD OF LIFE INSURANCE

Working for a life insurance company, I began looking at life expectancy very differently from the way I had as a practicing clinical physician. Your doctor cares deeply about you, and she hopes you live a long and healthy life. But her concern about your health pales when compared to a life insurance underwriter who has just insured your life for $1 million.

Your physician gets paid for finding and treating disease. Your life insurer is trying to group people according to their life expectancy, including a large group that is very healthy and going to live a very long time.

Who are these people who stand a good chance of reaching age 85 at a time when the average American is barely pushing 78—and smokers are averaging 71? This difference in life expectancy between unhealthy and healthy people is an astonishing 14 years!

Did you know that being obese or inactive has *the same impact* on life expectancy as smoking? Any of these three bad habits creates unhealthy people who suffer with more and longer illness, have a more difficult recovery, more and longer disability, and a shorter life.

IDENTIFYING THE HEALTHIEST GROUP OF PEOPLE

So if people who smoke, are overweight, or lead inactive lives have a much shorter life expectancy, who is in the group that lives seven years longer than average and lives a more illness-free life? And what do they do to stay so healthy?

This long-lived and very healthy group began to fascinate me. Just think of the tremendous benefits if you could identify and follow the habits and choices of the healthiest people. But identifying them is not enough unless you and I work together to plan how to follow these habits and choices. If we did, health care costs would plummet, chronic disease and disability would diminish, and greater numbers of people would live longer, healthier lives. The only losers would be the cardiologists, who would have less work to do—but I don't think we have to worry about them.

WHY DOES GETTING HEALTHY MATTER?

As I began to talk up making healthy choices to my friends and patients, I realized that while people found the information very interesting, they did not understand why any of this really mattered. So I started to give talks on preventing disease and promoting health. And after more than 50 presentations, television appearances, and media interviews, my ideas were ready to fit between the covers of a book.

Here's the message. Regardless of your current state of health, you can get healthier, and multiple studies have shown the simple steps you take to do it.

The simple answer to the question *Why does getting healthy matter?* is that it is far better to prevent a heart attack than to treat it well.

There are a myriad of diet and exercise and no-smoking books. I am not trying to compete with the how-to books. Rather, I want to show you how much bad health costs you, why good health matters, and how to get from one to the other. I hope to give you just enough scientific information to prove that you should try to be healthier. You should bother to make good health choices because you will live better, be sick less, have less disability, live longer, and be more active.

The good news is that you need to follow only seven basic prescriptions for really good health. So let's you and I get this discussion started. You'll learn the science supporting the benefits of healthy choices and how to make healthy choices, which will extend your life and improve its quality. You see, we are the first generation in history that can—and indeed must—plan on living with zest and vigor to age 85. But that's in chapter 3, and I'm getting ahead of myself.

Chapter 1

YOU ARE IN CONTROL

THE WIDENING HEALTH GAP

Most of us think we have little control over our future health—whether we have a heart attack at 68 or live vibrantly to 85. Nothing could be further from the truth. You control at least 70% of your own health.

How deeply ironic that science has identified the health habits that lead to a long life at the same time that the health of many people is threatened by tobacco, a sedentary lifestyle, obesity, and a surfeit of overly processed foods.

Most of us think there are only marginal health differences between choosing an inactive versus an active lifestyle or being obese versus being slender. Nothing could be further from the truth. The health differences between such groups are enormous. The people who make choices that undermine their health develop far more sickness, take longer to recover, spend many more health care dollars, and die sooner. The benefits to people who make good health choices include much better health by all measures—less illness, fewer heart attacks, less diabetes, less cancer, lower health care costs, and longer life.

WHAT DOES IT MEAN TO BE HEALTHY IN THE TWENTY-FIRST CENTURY?

We cannot rid the world of all illness. Many people live with illnesses such as asthma and psoriasis. These illnesses only rarely cause premature death. Some unlucky people will develop and die from an illness such as Parkinson's disease despite everything good they do in life. Fortunately, these illnesses are, in the overall scheme of things, relatively uncommon.

My focus in this book is on the very frequent and common chronic diseases that limit our good health. All of these share common causes. And the same lifestyle choices will prevent most of them.

The diseases that cause far and away the most illness, the most premature disabilities, and the most deaths include heart attacks, strokes, diabetes, cancers, and emphysema. While these illnesses may seem to happen the day they are diagnosed, in reality, they developed slowly as the direct result of individual lifestyle choices made over decades. These are the major diseases that limit our ability to live life to the fullest and the longest. These diseases are also largely preventable.

The healthiest people are those with the lowest risk of future disease. They have the fewest heart attacks, the lowest rate of diabetes, and the least cancer. They have the least disease, and if they are ill, they recover faster. They spend the fewest health care dollars. They have the most vigor and are the most active for the longest time. Healthy people may have illnesses such as asthma or psoriasis, but these do not interfere with their active life. They proactively make choices every day to minimize their risk of a chronic disease. This book describes what they do to stay so healthy.

An average person is at average risk for future disease. They float through life day to day without much regard for the future. Some will have a long life, others a shorter life, but they are not really trying to influence the outcome. They may know about and fear heart disease or diabetes, but their knowledge is incomplete. They are either blissfully ignorant of the steps they can take to prevent disease, or they are too involved elsewhere to pay attention to their health, or they are hopelessly confused by the mixed messages. Most average people pay attention to their health in a scattered and inconsistent manner. Every decade or so they decide to jog for a few months, but then they quit. They go on the low-fat diet this year and the low-carb diet next. They lose weight to win a bet with their friends. But they still eat cheesecake after the bet is won. Many average people are not aware how easily they can control their own future health. The average people are at an average risk for future serious disease.

Unhealthy people are those at the highest risk for premature death and disability. Whether intentional or not, they choose a lifestyle that significantly increases their risk of future disease. These people choose to smoke, or they choose to be very inactive, or they choose to eat large quantities of nutritionally poor food. They spend substantially more health care dollars than anyone else. By choosing this lifestyle for years on end, they substantially increase their risk of an early death.

Everyday Choices Do Matter

It's a fact: our everyday lifestyle choices and health habits directly influence whether we stay healthy or get a chronic disease such as diabetes, heart disease, or some cancers. The impact of these differences will be magnified as the huge baby boom generation lives long enough to see the final, long-term health result of their different lifestyles: premature disease or no disease.

Whether or not these diseases develop depends on the choices we and the boomers make every day. Take the stairs or ride the escalator? Eat unhealthy or healthy food? For example, will you eat a crisp apple or a fast-food apple pie as a midafternoon snack? One will give you a ton of disease-fighting phytochemicals, flavonoids, antioxidants, and fiber. The other will give a tiny little bit of fruit and a whole lot of disease-causing, deep-fried, highly processed simple sugars. The impact of such choices is additive, cumulative, and synergistic—bettering or eroding your health.

Since each health choice you or I make acts either as a plus or a minus, placing us above or below the health "average," the impact of these many decisions can be huge when piled up over a lifetime. Each time you choose, you are stockpiling the effects of either right or wrong health decisions.

If you are a healthy person, more often than not, you have developed a habit of making consistently healthy choices. And you make a healthy and informed choice in *all* of the seven important areas, not in just one. You do not smoke but you do eat broccoli, take a 30-minute walk every day, and take medication to control your high blood pressure every day. Your informed choices can keep you healthy for today as well as prevent the development of chronic disease tomorrow.

Unhealthy people consistently make unhealthy choices. They may choose to smoke, lead inactive lives, eat a steady diet of convenience foods, or eat too much. These people do not understand the real damage they are doing to their health. Adding one bad health choice on top of another for decades does more than undermine their good health. These habits actually promote illness.

If you have made some unhealthy choices, you are not alone. A very large and growing number of people are right there with you. At least 25% of Americans smoke tobacco, another 30% meet the federal definition of obesity, and 60% are sedentary or do so little exercise it does not count.

Fortunately, our bodies are wonderfully forgiving and have the ability to heal. If you have made a lifetime of wrong health choices, you can still recover and attain good health. If you quit smoking, your body will begin to heal within hours. If you are inactive, you can get physically fit and strong. If you are obese, you can lose weight. If you ate too many doughnuts and chips, your body will welcome a new regimen of health-promoting fruits and vegetables and whole grains. All of these healthy choices will decrease your risk of future disease.

Dr. Bob promises:

◆ *You are never too old or too ill to start a healthier life.*

It does not matter where you are now or where you are coming from. The only thing that matters is where you are going. The positive effect of making healthy choices is immense and worth more than any effort you expend.

WHAT THE STUDIES SHOW ABOUT THE HEALTHIEST PEOPLE

Healthy people have been analyzed in several large epidemiological studies (studies that investigate the spread, prevention, and control of disease). Specialists followed large groups of people over several years. These groups, such as those in the Seven Countries Study, the Iowa Women's Health Study, the Physicians' Health Study, the Multiple Risk Factor Intervention Trial, the Honolulu Heart Study, and the Okinawa Centenarian Study, have provided insights into the habits of people with very good health, health that is substantially better than average.

Medical researchers have identified the daily habits of men and women with substantially less heart disease, diabetes, and cancer. These people live longer and healthier lives than everyone else. They have less illness, less disability, and spend fewer health care dollars.

Researchers have found that the health habits of the healthiest people are largely consistent among studies and across cultures. You can adopt all of these health habits with a little knowledge and guidance.

Interestingly, the same good habits prevent most of the chronic degenerative diseases, including heart attacks, peripheral vascular disease, stroke, type 2 diabetes, obesity, and many cancers. And the most recent research indicates these same good habits may reduce the risk of Alzheimer's Disease.

The daily health habits that these people practice with such good results form the seven prescriptions for healthy living contained in this book.

BEING HEALTHY

Healthy people are not just people lucky enough to be born with good genes. Healthy people understand that preventing a heart attack is far better than treating it well. Their lifestyle habits are not difficult or expensive. They do not require spandex, a membership in the fitness center, or a restrictive diet. The health habits that promote good health are astonishingly simple and work together in a positive way.

These differences between health-promoting and disease-promoting choices are simpler, clearer, and more powerful than originally thought. Healthy people often have subtly different ways of living, exercising, and eating than nonhealthy people. For healthy people, these differences lead to a vastly better future.

Understanding the implications of these differences can change our understanding of what it means to be older. John Rowe, M.D., and Robert Kahn, Ph.D., published *Successful Aging*,[1] a very readable book that summarizes the famous MacArthur Foundation Study on Aging. The authors note that the adverse effects of the aging process on mobility and strength have been exaggerated. They emphasize that adopting a healthy diet, exercise, personal habits, and psychosocial factors (such as a loving spouse, good friends, and a job you like) can lessen many age-related losses. They could not be more correct.

Dr. Bob promises:

◆ *Everyone can choose to live a long, vibrant life filled with vim and vigor. You'll feel better, look more attractive, be stronger, and live longer.*

◆ *You are closer to good health than you realize.*

◆ *Small changes in your daily routines can and will make a big change in your health and future.*

◆ *The choices that result in good health are simple. They are not difficult or complex. No special gimmicks, diets, pills, supplements, or regimens are required.*

◆ *Neither chronic disease nor the previously assumed "natural decline with aging" is inevitable. In fact, you can have a very active life for a long time with few limitations and much less disease.*

So how can you join the healthiest people on the path to the best health? How can you make the same choices as these healthy people? What benefit can you gain from following their good health habits? And what can you and I—the somewhat sedentary, out-of-shape, and overweight people who eat the wrong diet—do to join the healthy?

The choices below seem simple, but done consistently and all together, they give you a very healthy life.

Dr. Bob's seven prescriptions:

1. Choose not to smoke.

2. Choose to get 30 minutes of moderate physical activity every day.

3. Choose to maintain a healthy weight.

4. Choose to eat reasonable portion sizes, including five or more servings of colorful fruits and vegetables, nuts and two whole grains daily; fish twice a week; cook with monounsaturated and polyunsaturated oils, like olive or soybean oils.

5. Choose to drink modest amounts of alcohol if you drink at all.

6. Choose to unwind; be kind to yourself.

7. Choose to work with your physician to prevent disease.

Choose wisely to live well and to live long.

Test Your Health IQ

The short ten-question quiz below will help you understand why you should read this book.

1. How many more years of life will a healthy, nonsmoking 60-year-old live?
   a. 10 years
   b. 15 years
   c. 20 years
   d. 25 years

2. How many current 60-year-olds will live to age 100?
   a. 0.1%
   b. 1%
   c. 3%
   d. 5%

3. Heart disease kills more than _____ Americans per year.
    a. 100,000
    b. 250,000
    c. 750,000
    d. 1,000,000

4. Heart disease kills more women than the next ___ causes of death combined.
    a. 1
    b. 3
    c. 7
    d. 14

5. Which activity or activities double your chance of dying?
    a. Smoking
    b. Obesity
    c. Getting no exercise
    d. Uncontrolled hypertension
    e. Cholesterol over 300
    f. All of the above

6. What percentage of your physical health is under your control?
    a. 20%
    b. 30%
    c. 50%
    d. 70%

7. Compare the size of the average American today with the average American of 1970.
    a. The same
    b. Only slightly larger
    c. Significantly larger

8. Compare the average number of calories eaten every day with the number eaten 20 years ago.
   a. The same
   b. 2% or 3% more
   c. 10% more
   d. 15% more

9. Eating a diet high in fruits, vegetables, whole grains, fish, nuts, and plant-based (liquid) oils, but low in saturated and trans-fatty acids will reduce your risk of heart disease and cancer by how much?
   a. Not at all
   b. 5%
   c. 15%
   d. More than 30%

10. For each mile walked per week, the average death rate decreases by what percent?
    a. Negligible
    b. 1%
    c. 4%
    d. 10%

ANSWERS:

1. d. The very healthy, nonsmoking 60-year-old will live another 25 years.

2. d. 5% of current 60-year-olds will live to 100. The future centenarians of 2050 are alive today. Many of us will be among them.

3. c. Heart disease, the leading cause of death in America today, kills more than 750,000 Americans each year. What's more, heart disease was the leading cause of death every year of the 20th century except for the 1918 flu epidemic. Heart disease causes more deaths, in both men and women, than the next five leading causes of death combined. The tragedy is that heart disease is a preventable disease.

4. c. Heart disease kills more women than the next seven causes of death combined. Heart disease kills more than 10 times as many women as breast cancer.

5 f. Your chances of dying in a given year double if you smoke or are obese or inactive or have uncontrolled hypertension or a very high cholesterol.

6. d. You control 70% of your own health. The everyday choices you make are important and do determine your health.

7. c. More Americans are significantly more obese today than ever before.

8. c. Americans eat 300 more calories today than in 1975. Every added 3,500 calories becomes one more pound. It is a wonder we do not all weigh more.

9. d. Eating a healthy diet can reduce your risk of heat disease at least 30%. Colorful fruits and vegetables, whole grains, nuts, fish, and plant-based oils are all health-promoting foods.

10. c. For each mile walked consistently per week, the risk of heart disease falls 4%. Walking briskly is one of the best and simplest exercises that every person can do.

Chapter 2

YOU CHOOSE
YOUR OWN HEALTH

You control far more of your personal health than you think. And this control is far more important than you think. You can choose to lead a lifestyle that causes obesity and weakness and that raises your risk of heart disease, diabetes, and cancer—all of which lead to an early and prolonged period of disability and premature death. Or, by making better everyday choices, you can live a relatively disease-free and active life with minimal periods of sickness and disability, even though you live longer.

Regardless of your current state of health, you can get healthier. Your body is capable of tremendous healing that begins as soon as your destructive behavior stops and your healthy habits begin. Even 30 years of neglect can be reversed quite quickly. It's all a matter of the choices you make. If you quit smoking, the health benefits start within 24 hours after you quit and continue to increase for 10 years. If you are weak, exercise can make you strong. By switching from an unhealthy to a healthy diet, you can slow or stop the progression of heart disease. You can prevent diabetes by choosing to be active and lose weight.

You Control 70% of Your Own Health

Many of us think our genes or environmental toxins determine our health—and we're banking on modern medicine to come to our rescue. In fact, just the opposite is true. You control as much as 70% of your own health, disability, and longevity. The healthiest people who consistently make a lifetime of healthy choices live longer and with fewer medical problems than the people who fail to make good health choices.

Science Has Proven This

The Nurses' Health Study[2] has looked in detail at the daily lives of more than 85,000 nurses for more than 20 years. This study recently identified a group of women who had only 20% of the risk of heart attack compared to all other women in the study. These healthy women had all made simple choices for good health. There were no secrets, difficult exercises, or costly dietary supplements. Among the healthiest nurses, the best long-term health came from five simple choices made in their basic, everyday living. These women:

1. did not smoke,

2. exercised moderately at least 30 minutes most days of the week,

3. maintained a normal body weight defined as a BMI (body mass index) less than 25 (see chapter 6 for an explanation of BMI),

4. ate a diet high in fruits, vegetables, cereal fiber, and a high polyunsaturated-to-saturated fat ratio (i.e., liquid to animal fat),

5. drank the equivalent of 1 teaspoon of alcohol a day.

You have to admit, this is not a complicated list. The data show these five health choices reduce heart disease, diabetes, and cancer. Following these choices affects when we become ill and determines what happens to us at the end of life.

In another important long-term study, Dr. Anthony Vita[3] studied 1,750 university graduates until their average age was 75. He classified participants into high-, moderate-, and low-risk groups based on their smoking, exercise patterns, and body mass index (see chapter 6). The people in the high-risk group spent twice as much time disabled or ill as those in the low-risk group. In addition, the low-risk group deferred the onset of disability by more than five years. The conclusion is clear: people with better health habits live longer and any disability they experience is compressed into fewer years at the very end of life.

This is a very strong statement, with an easily understood bottom line: do not smoke, but make time to exercise and maintain a healthy weight to enjoy a longer, more active life with less disability.

Multiple studies have underscored similar important research findings. Some of the best information on the importance and value of personal choices comes from several studies of huge segments of the population now under way: the Nurses' Health Study, the Physicians' Health Study, the Iowa Women's Health Study, and the Multiple Risk Factor Intervention Trial. These decades-long studies of thousands of people nationwide have repeatedly and strongly demonstrated the impact and importance that personal choice plays in determining health. The evidence is overwhelming.

As a careful reader you may note some inconsistencies in the numbers of people involved in the large epidemiological studies. These differences occur because some study subjects did not qualify for or complete all parts of the study.

Your Health Is Not All in Your Genes

Genetics certainly has a lot to do with our health, but probably not as much as you might think. For certain, there are a very few lucky people who inherit a gene for exceptional longevity. Likewise, there are a few unlucky people who inherit a gene for the early onset of a dread disease, such as muscular dystrophy. However, both of these occurrences are the rare exceptions to the rule. Most of us are somewhere in the middle.

Do your genes spell out your health destiny? On one hand, the genes you inherited from your parents control everything from the color of your eyes, to your height, and some of your risk for heart disease. On the other hand—and with few exceptions—you largely influence how your genes affect you. While you may not be able to change your eye color, you can control whether or not the genes that put you at risk for heart disease result in premature disease or good health.

Understanding your family health risk is essential to avoid history repeating itself. If colon cancer runs in your family, you need to recognize that you may have inherited this same risk. Armed with this knowledge, you can then take the steps to prevent the same fate.

Knowing you have a family history of premature heart disease is a wake-up call. There may be as many as 100 or more genes that interact with one another to produce or prevent heart disease. Medical scientists may not yet understand the genetics of heart disease, but they do understand the biochemistry leading to hardening of the arteries (or atherosclerosis) and heart disease. Physicians can identify who is at risk and prevent atherosclerosis and heart attacks. Today a family history of premature heart disease need not condemn you to the same fate.

John, now age 54, grew up in a family that seemed to meet every few years for the funeral of another male relative. As John remembered it, his father, two of three paternal uncles, and his older brother all either had their first heart attack or died by age 53. John was 50 when he visited his brother in the coronary care unit. Up until then, John had played the tough guy, laughing off the family history. He had never smoked, but outside of not smoking, John didn't think he could do very much to prevent "the inevitable."

At the urging of his wife and mother, John made an appointment for a physical with a preventive cardiologist. At the time of the first exam, John weighed 248 pounds and stood 6'1". His EKG and treadmill electrocardiogram were normal. But his total cholesterol was very high at 270; his "bad" LDL cholesterol was very high at 180; and his "good" HDL cholesterol was very low at 34. His blood pressure was elevated at 142/94. However, along with the bad news, John also learned that he could make choices to prevent heart disease and that he could reduce his risk.

John started medications to lower his blood pressure and improve his cholesterol. He began a program of diet and exercise. Understanding that he could do something about his risk was his prime motivator, and he stuck to his diet and exercise plan.

Three years later, John walks five days a week for 30 to 60 minutes a day at 4 miles an hour, plays racquetball or tennis weekly, follows a diet that is high in fruits and vegetables, eats fish a couple of times per week, eats whole grains, and uses olive oil when he cooks. He limits saturated fats (such as premium ice cream) and avoids commercially prepared foods as much as possible. He takes a medication to lower his cholesterol and a blood pressure pill with excellent results.

He still stands 6'1", but now he weighs 184 pounds. John's blood pressure is very good—126/74. His total cholesterol is now normal at 176, as are his LDL at 98 and his HDL at 44. His EKG and treadmill are normal. He walked for 15 full minutes on the treadmill, an excellent time demonstrating his excellent fitness.

Best of all, he received a good health endorsement from his life insurance company. For his 53rd birthday, he bought more life insurance and received the lowest possible price rating. The company's underwriter put him into a large group of people with an average life expectancy of 80 years. Not bad for a man who once thought he might be dead at 53.

The same power of prevention exists even with some kinds of familial cancer. For example, recognizing you were born into a family with lots of early colon cancer gives you an opportunity to prevent the disease. Inherited colon cancer is almost totally preventable with effective cancer screening. Embarrassing, yes, a little. Effective, totally—with minimal risk but moderate cost. The value of regular screening to prevent the disease in people with a family history of colon cancer is incredible. Effective colon cancer screening should be able to virtually eliminate the disease within a decade.

Your Health Is Largely the Result of Toxins, Just Not the Toxins You Think

Genetic fatalism is one misconception people have about their health. Here's another: many people think that their health is seriously damaged by environmental toxins. They fear the pollutants in the air they breathe and pesticides in the food they eat. They are correct to a point but not to the extent they imagine.

True, our air could be cleaner, and pollution does cause asthma and other respiratory problems. However, the surest way to improve the public's respiratory health is to ban all smoking outright. Cigarette smoke injures your lungs more than the pollutants your car gives off. If we banned smoking, both the smoker's bronchitis and the asthmatic who breathes the secondhand smoke would improve immediately.

No one wants pesticides in their drinking water. Everyone wants organic food straight from the backyard. But even backyard gardeners often use pesticides to kill the bugs that eat tomatoes, corn, beans, and lettuce. The truth of the matter is that the health benefits you get from eating fruits and vegetables far outweigh any potential harm from pesticides.

Don't get me wrong here—I am all in favor of a cleaner environment and organic food. Keeping the environment as clean as possible benefits us all. Keeping our food safe and clean is critical.

However, if you want to focus on toxins, the really scary toxins are those we most often overlook. They lurk in your cupboard and on store shelves. I am talking about the man-made chemicals in your food as well as the kinds of foods you eat. The highly processed, sugared servings of partially hydrogenated fats we know as candy bars or snack foods are a health disaster. The junk food you eat damages your health far more than the pesticides on your grapes.

What environmental chemicals should you worry about? How about the saturated fats in those French fries? How about trans-fatty acids, those partially hydrogenated fats used to make store-bought cookies and found in deep-fat fryers? These fats are, without a doubt, harmful to your arteries, yet many of us willingly eat a couple of pounds of them every year. How about the sugars and high-fructose corn syrup used to sweeten most everything today? Some children get 20% of their total daily calories from sugars and high-fructose corn syrup, a product that barely existed 25 years ago. Some children today eat 30 teaspoons of refined sugar per day in sodas, snacks, and candy.[4]

YOUR HEALTH ACCUMULATES OVER DECADES, FOR BETTER OR WORSE

While knowing that you are responsible for 70% of your own health is good news, it is also a bit daunting. Before this, you may have thought that genetics and the environment shaped your health. Not so. Your health is the result of the small decisions that you make all day long. They accumulate over days and decades. Those seemingly insignificant choices, such as what size popcorn to have at the movies and whether to take the stairs or the elevator, determine your health.

Don't be lulled into thinking that great health is the result of a miracle. Rather, great health comes from *consistently* making healthier choices over a lifetime.

Dr. Bob says:

♦ *Great health does not mean that you have to be perfect. Great health comes from making the correct health choice more often than not for your whole life.*

And on the other side of the coin, bad luck only rarely causes bad health. More commonly, it is the result of consistently making unhealthy choices. Most major diseases today are chronic degenerative diseases that took decades of consistently bad choices to develop: years and years in which you chose to smoke, or didn't bother to control your weight, or sat around more than you moved, or consistently ate highly processed convenience foods and junk foods. Those are the choices that caused the heart attack.

Your arteries do not harden just because you ate one bacon cheeseburger or smoked one cigarette or nibbled a few too many chocolate-chip cookies. Arteries harden after decades of smoking, a steady intake of bacon double cheeseburgers with fries, or thousands of chocolate-chip cookies. Your health is not the result of any one choice on any given day. Yes, you can eat a doughnut. Yes, you can take the elevator. Yes, you can watch television. You just cannot eat three donuts and watch four hours of television every day.

What's more, your health is not the result of being virtuous in one area and neglecting everything else healthy. You cannot be healthy if you are a marathon runner but you smoke. (Yes, such people do exist.) You cannot be healthy if you are a thin, healthy eater but do not exercise.

Ron never worried about his health. He always told everyone that he would worry about his health when it ran out. Ron joked that he needed to keep a few bad habits in reserve so he had something to give up when he had a heart attack.

Ron took up cigars when he could no longer smoke in the office. He smoked 10 or 12 cigars a week, and he inhaled more than a little.

Ron "exercised" a couple of times a week. He would go to the health club, where he read the morning paper while strolling on the treadmill. He would spend some time in the steam room and then cool off in the lounge before returning to the office. The gym gave Ron an opportunity to visit with everyone just as he did on the golf course. In reality, his channel-changing thumb was the best-exercised muscle in his body. Ron loved anything that made life easier: golf carts, escalators, moving sidewalks, four-wheel drive vehicles so he could park closer to his cabin—climbing up that hill was murder!

Sure, he had put on a generous 60 pounds since college, but his tailor, a diplomatic fellow, called Ron "stocky," which he took as a compliment. Airplane seats felt snugger than they used to, but certainly that wasn't because of anything Ron did. Besides, Ron knew several people who were a whole lot heavier than he was. Therefore, Ron decided he did not have a weight problem.

Ron's diet was nearly 100% unhealthy. Breakfast was either just coffee, or coffee with a lumberjack special: a three-egg omelet with cheese, potatoes, sausage, and at least one sweet roll. Juice, oatmeal, and fruit never made it to Ron's table.

He had a knack for making his lunch look better than anyone else's, maybe because he could sweet-talk even the most hardened waiter or waitress into layering an extra inch of pastrami onto his sandwich. No one could understand why his bacon cheeseburgers always looked better than everyone else's, although some suspected he tipped the cook at the nineteenth hole. Dinner? Tossed iceberg lettuce with blue cheese dressing, steak or fried chicken, mashed potatoes, and if he was lucky, chocolate cake with "just a little ice cream—have to watch the diet, you know."

Ron's idea of a green vegetable was the pickle on his cheeseburger. What about whole grains? The sesame seeds on his hamburger bun. Seafood? A Friday-night fish fry.

After 30 years of eating like this, Ron thought he was in "okay shape," a little overweight but pretty much able to do everything he still wanted to do. To make absolutely certain that he did not have any medical problems, he simply did not go to the doctor. This was Ron's idea of prevention: avoid the doctor and so avoid any bad news. After all, why would he want to find out he had to give up a bad habit prematurely? Besides, he knew that doctors were getting really good at treating heart attacks, weren't they?

You probably know several people like Ron. He is the prime example of an unhealthy person who consistently makes poor lifestyle choices. He just isn't feeling the effect yet. His smoking has not caused noticeable shortness of breath. Ron is still young enough and strong enough to do what he wants. His extra weight has not yet caused diabetes. His diet, smoking, and inactivity may have caused some hardening of the arteries, but nothing severe enough to cause a heart attack—yet. Someday Ron will go to the doctor, one way or the other.

The real questions for Ron are:

1. What is so wrong with the way he lives?

2. Why should Ron care?

3. If Ron changes his lifestyle to make healthier choices, will he have to eat tofu and run marathons?

And the answers are:

1. Ron may like his lifestyle, but by making consistently unhealthy choices, he is dramatically increasing his risk of premature disease.

2. Ron should care because right now he is headed straight for the early onset of chronic disease and a premature death. If he chooses to change his habits, his body will start to recover. He can significantly decrease his risk of future disease by changing *now*.

3. No, Ron will not have to eat tofu or run at all. The choices for good health are not unpleasant or difficult. And they do not require the added expense of an exercise gym or special foods.

We have all been lulled into complacency by an enabling society, one that has told us that it's okay to eat too much of all the wrong foods, that we do not need to exercise, that modern medicine will take care of us. We are invited to avoid even the simple activities and exercises of daily life. But the truth is that our past bills are close to coming due, and we, like Ron, must determine our own health future. Technology and modern medicine will not rescue us from this one. We have to make the choice to change on our own.

Your Money and Your Health

Good health planning is like good financial planning. Both require that you make informed choices and follow a course of action. Both pay long-term dividends.

We all know the basic rules for saving money so we have enough for both today and retirement. You start with an overall financial plan: pay your tax-free retirement accounts first, spend less than you earn, diversify your investments, and invest wisely for the long term. Over time, and because of the wonders of compound tax-deferred interest, your daily savings grow into a million-dollar retirement fund. You know you cannot fund your retirement by making one or two lump-sum payments a few months before you retire.

The steps for your good health are just like a good financial plan. You start by deciding to be healthy. You choose to not smoke, to get regular exercise, to maintain a normal weight, and to eat well. You make little choices every day. You are investing in these good health choices, and the return on your investment is to enjoy the best health later on. Because you are continually taking good care of your health, your health improves over time. As you age, you are able to continue your active and vigorous life.

Where Do You Want to Be in Twenty Years?

As we look to our future, we should be depositing good health choices as well as saving for retirement, so that we may enjoy excellent health along with the leisure our money brings us. No one wants to find themselves with both poor health and inadequate financial resources. Very few people want good health and not enough money or poor health and good money. We all want both good health and enough money to last forever. Table 1 below explains our choices.

	Poor health	Excellent health
Table 1 YOUR MONEY AND YOUR HEALTH		
Inadequate money	Poor health and no money	Excellent health but no money
More than adequate money	Poor health but more than enough money	Excellent health and more than enough money

This table shows everyone's goal of wanting both good health and enough money. Which corner are you headed for?

GOOD HEALTH IS LOST IN THE MEDIA DETAILS

The media inundates us with mixed messages about better health. The messages seem complex, overly scientific, and out of reach. They are also contradictory: Do you need to be a marathon-running vegetarian, or can you be healthy with moderate exercise and a sensible diet? Should I be on a high-fat or a no-fat diet? How much fat should be in a low-carb diet? And what, pray tell, is a "net carb"?

Nearly everyone talks about their diet, the food on their plate, the food they didn't put on their plate, whether they are on Atkins, the South Beach, the grapefruit, or the ultra-low-fat diet. They talk about the exercise program they've started or the program they didn't start. The media keeps up a constant drumbeat of new diets, trendy exercise programs, New Year's resolutions, foods to eat and foods to avoid, and new scientific studies to support today's hot topic. Science keeps pumping out new studies that slightly contradict the preceding study. Merchants push, peddle, and press the newest piece of exercise equipment or pill to keep us all young and sexy.

The message of good health is lost in these contradictory studies and details. Any hope of change is sacrificed to the despair of not knowing which health message to believe.

Choose to Make Good Health Happen

In reality, good health is deceptively close and simple. Good health is within all of us. *Given the opportunity, your body can begin to heal itself.* However, you have to help your body: by choosing to give up unhealthy habits and by making good and healthy choices. Healthy choices have tremendous power to heal and prevent disease.

Following my seven prescriptions—or even aiming at them—can significantly improve your health. You are removing a bad health choice and replacing it with a good health choice. All of us need to start making these choices, trading an unhealthy for a healthy option. These trades enable our bodies to heal themselves and resist the diseases that modern life promotes.

Dr. Bob promises:

◆ *The change for good health is definitely worth any effort you put into it.*

Make no mistake: it takes a lot of courage even to think about eating better and getting in shape, let alone going to a fitness club. In our busy lives, it takes courage to find or make the time. The purpose of this book is to draw a very straight path that cuts through all of the hype and hoopla, a straight path to better health within a time schedule that fits into your day. The path is not very sexy or flashy, but it is certainly true. Follow this path, and you will end at a much healthier place.

You are closer to good health than you know. The most difficult step of any journey is the first one. The Buddhists say it so well: "Start where you are." Get rid of the guilt. Overcome your inertia. Just make today a healthier day than yesterday and tomorrow healthier than today. Add a little walk here, skip the chips there, enjoy some salmon and a glass of wine for dinner, have an orange for dessert.

The past is history. You are at a place called now and today. Today I'm writing your first prescription for better health.

Dr. Bob's says:

◆ *Make today healthier than yesterday was—even if it's only slightly healthier.*

Your first step may be small, but it's a first step down a path that will alter your life. Then keep making tomorrow healthier than today.

Chapter 3

LIVING WELL, MAYBE EVEN TO AGE 100

Just how long will you live? In 19 of the past 20 centuries of human history, life expectancy increased at the rate of one more year of life for every century. This changed about 100 years ago. Over the last century alone, life expectancy has increased 30 years due to major advances in sanitation and improvements in medical science. Table 2 gives you a quick look at life expectancy throughout history. It shows just how radically we are extending our lives.

To be sure, in every century, some people lived to a very old age. The new change is that now many more people are living to old age. In fact, everyone must assume and plan for their own old age.

	Table 2	
Changes in life expectancy over the past 2,000 years		
Famous Event	Year	Average Life Expectancy from Birth
Julius Caesar dies	44 BC	22
US Declaration of Independence signed	1776	35
Bismarck of Germany declares 65 to be the age of retirement	1889	48
Turn of last century	1900	48
WW I ends	1917	51
Stock market crashes	1929	57
First baby boomers born	1946	66
President Kennedy assassinated	1963	69
Y2K did not happen	2000	78

Life expectancy continues even now to increase, but most likely at a slightly slower rate of increase than 50 years ago. Plotted on a graph, this is what the dramatic change in life expectancy looks like:

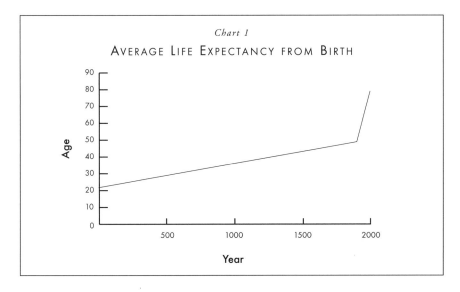

Specifically, what accounts for people living longer during the last century?

1. Public health has substantially improved—we have safer drinking water, refrigerated foods, better housing, sanitation, and sewage control.

2. Medical science has nearly eliminated infant and premature deaths from infectious disease.

3. Since 1960, the number of smokers has substantially declined from nearly 50% to 25% of the population.

4. Heart-related deaths have fallen off nearly 50% in the past 40 years.

Given all of these advances, we now live long enough to reap the results of our personal lifestyle choices: good health or disease. That fact should make us all sit up and take notice.

So here's a mind shift for you: you will probably live much longer than you think. That means, barring fatal accidents, you'll live long enough that any bad health habits you've practiced over the years will catch up with you. On the other hand, if you heed the seven prescriptions contained in this book, you will be much more likely to enjoy that longer life, free of the maladies usually associated with aging.

Here's a theme of this book: *aging is a process, not a disease.* If you do it right—make healthy choices all along the way—it is biologically possible to grow old without disease. We can all live long lives with great vigor, vitality, and vibrancy.

LIVING TO A VERY OLD AGE

The very fact you have survived life this far means that you can expect to live longer than the 78 years predicted for you at birth. In fact, once you reach age 55, you can—and must—plan on living to age 80, or even 85. A substantial number of us will live longer than 90. Choosing good health will matter more than you think.

Some demographers are even wondering if we should plan on living to 100. The United Nations population predictions show that 1 in 20 baby boomers might reach 100 "thanks to breakthroughs in treatment for heart disease and cancer, lives relatively free of hard labor, and long-standing memberships at the gym."[5] Clearly, these healthy centenarians will come from those who choose good health all along the path of their lives.

Today, 70,000 centenarians are alive in America. By the year 2050, that number will grow to somewhere between 800,000 and 4 million. The U.S. Census Bureau officially estimates that 1.1 million Americans will be centenarians in 2050.[6]

While it may take some time to get used to the idea you might live to 100, it is not something to be feared. Centenarians spend the least amount of money on health care, they are often surprisingly independent, they tend to experience minimal disability, and they often die relatively quickly after a short illness.

To paraphrase the comic strip character Pogo, "We have met the centenarian and he is us."

Let's step back a moment to remind ourselves that simply living to a very old age is not the goal. *The goal is to live the longest, most active life with the fewest limitations possible.* This book tells you how to do that—how to maximize your chances to live most actively for the longest possible time. It all centers on minimizing your risk for premature disease.

WHAT THE NUMBERS SAY ABOUT THE IMPORTANCE OF CHOOSING GOOD HEALTH

Actuaries are mathematicians who study life expectancy and rates of death. Understanding their view of the world will illustrate the differences between average, good, and bad health and show how these health differences affect us. This next section looks at a very simplified view of life and death as seen by an actuary working in the insurance industry.

Table 3 shows the *average* number of years of life remaining and life expectancy assuming that a person has survived to the age in the far left column. As the graph shows, according to the 2000 U.S. Vital Statistics, having survived to age 65, the *average* American man may expect to live another 16.1 years to age 81 and a woman 19.1 years to age 84.[7]

Table 3

AVERAGE YEARS OF LIFE REMAINING AND LIFE EXPECTANCY
FOR A GIVEN AGE AND SEX

Source: 2000 U.S. Vital Statistics.

Age	Male		Female	
	Years of life remaining	Life expectancy	Years of life remaining	Life expectancy
0	73.9	73.9	79.4	79.4
10	64.7	74.7	70.1	80.1
20	55.0	75.0	60.2	80.2
30	45.7	75.7	50.5	80.5
40	36.5	76.5	41.0	81.0
50	27.7	77.7	31.7	81.7
60	19.6	79.6	23.1	83.1
65	16.1	81.1	19.1	84.1
70	12.8	82.8	15.4	85.4
80	7.5	87.5	9.1	89.1
90	4.1	94.1	4.8	94.8
100	2.4	102.4	2.7	102.7

Life expectancy tables are published by the Department of Vital Statistics of the United States, the IRS, and the Society of Actuaries. Life insurance premiums, Social Security, pension, and annuity payouts all rely on this important data.

The important word in table 3 is "average." "Average" includes everyone. It does not differentiate among marathon-running vegetarians, smokers, and hospice patients. Talking about average life expectancy masks individual differences.

Actuaries study these differences by analyzing the number of deaths expected to occur for groups of 1,000 people of the same age and with similar characteristics.[8] As you look at table 4, understand that

1. some deaths occur at every age;

2. deaths become more frequent as we get older;

3. people who smoke, those with a high risk for disease, or those with a disease such as heart disease are more likely than others to die in a given year.[9]

Table 4 shows the expected number of deaths for a group of 1,000 people of that given age. The number of annual deaths in this kind of table is based on 1,000 in each starting age group. For example, in a group of 1,000 women, each age 60, actuaries expect 7.7 will die next year. The following year when the women are 61, the actuary would start a new group with 1,000 to find the expected number of deaths for the following year. This data gives the same life expectancy by age used in table 3.

Table 4

NUMBER OF EXPECTED DEATHS PER 1,000 PER YEAR FOR THE AVERAGE
MAN AND WOMAN OF A GIVEN AGE (AGES ROUNDED)

Source: National Vital Statistics Reports, Vol. 51, No. 5, March 14, 2003.

	Male	Female
Age	Average population	Average population
1	8.06	6.63
10	0.21	0.15
20	1.15	0.43
30	1.39	0.64
40	2.55	1.43
50	5.43	3.13
60	12.31	7.7
70	29.80	19.21
80	69.73	48.15
Over 85	175.01	147.19

Like all averages, the average life expectancy includes some
people who live fewer years and others who live more years around
the average. Several known health factors can move a person above
or below the average. Let's look at some.

THE GROUP THAT DOESN'T REACH AVERAGE AGE

People who smoke live fewer years than nonsmokers. The
question for an actuary is, when do these deaths occur? The answer
is that they occur all along the course of life.

In the mid-1960s, life insurers began reflecting the mortality difference between smokers and nonsmokers in the price of insurance premiums. The mortality difference has increased since then and is now more than double that of nonsmokers.[10] This doubling of expected deaths per year at every age means that smokers can count on dying seven years earlier than average nonsmokers.

Obesity, defined here as a BMI over 30 (see chapter 6), and a sedentary life shorten life expectancy as much as smoking,[11] which means that these lifestyle choices also double the risk of death at every age. Table 5 shows the effect of this doubling of the number of expected deaths per year.

Table 5

NUMBER OF EXPECTED DEATHS PER 1,000 PER YEAR FOR THE AVERAGE AND WORSE-THAN-AVERAGE MAN AND WOMAN OF A GIVEN AGE

Age	Male		Female	
	Average population from table 4	Smoking or obesity or sedentary lifestyle doubles the risk of death	Average population from table 4	Smoking or obesity or sedentary lifestyle doubles the risk of death
1	8.06	*	6.63	*
1–4	0.36	*	0.29	*
5–14	0.21	*	0.15	*
15–24	1.15	2.30	0.43	0.86
25–34	1.39	2.78	0.64	1.28
35–44	2.55	5.10	1.43	2.86
45–54	5.43	10.86	3.13	6.26
55–64	12.31	24.62	7.70	15.40
65–74	29.80	59.60	19.21	38.42
75–84	69.73	139.46	48.15	96.30
> 85	175.01	**	147.19	**

* Not given because too few smokers under age 15.

** Not given because number of people meeting higher risk criteria here deemed too small.

THE GROUP THAT OUTLIVES THE AVERAGE

We have just identified how death increases at all ages among unhealthy people compared to the *average*. Now let's look at the people who live longer than the average. In order to have an average, you must have a group made up of an equal number of people who live an equal number of years longer than average. So what does the expected death rate look like for a group that is going to live to age 85?

As you might guess, these healthy people have a substantially lower number of expected deaths per 1,000 than the average group. And a whole lot fewer deaths than the unhealthy people.

These healthy people have a low risk for heart disease, cancer, and diabetes. Why? They do not smoke. They exercise daily, maintain a normal weight, eat health-promoting foods, control stress, and see their physician about preventive medical care. Several recent large studies, discussed in greater detail later in the book, have demonstrated that these healthy lifestyle choices can reduce disease and disability and increase longevity.

Table 6 below compares the expected deaths for a healthy group to the average and worse-than-average death rates. In order to reach an average life expectancy of age 85, the death rates at each age must decline by 50%. The astonishing result is that the healthy group has half of the expected deaths per 1,000 per year as the average people and one quarter of the deaths of the unhealthy group.

Table 6

NUMBER OF EXPECTED DEATHS PER 1,000 PER YEAR FOR THE BETTER-THAN-AVERAGE, AVERAGE, AND WORSE-THAN-AVERAGE MAN AND WOMAN OF A GIVEN AGE

	Expected number of deaths per 1,000 per year					
	Male			Female		
	Best health lifestyle reduces risk of death by half	Average population (from table 4 above)	Smoking or obesity or sedentary lifestyle (from table 5 above)	Best health lifestyle reduces risk of death by half	Average population (from table 4 above)	Smoking or obesity or sedentary lifestyle (from table 5 above)
Age						
15–24	0.57	1.15	2.30	0.22	0.43	0.86
25–34	0.69	1.39	2.78	0.62	0.64	1.28
35–44	1.27	2.55	5.10	0.72	1.43	2.86
45–54	2.22	5.43	10.86	1.56	3.13	6.26
55–64	6.15	12.31	24.62	3.85	7.70	15.40
65–74	14.90	29.80	59.60	9.61	19.21	38.42
75–84	34.86	69.73	139.46	24.07	48.15	96.30

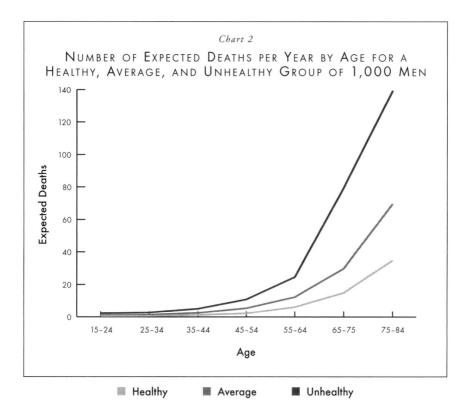

Chart 2

NUMBER OF EXPECTED DEATHS PER YEAR BY AGE FOR A
HEALTHY, AVERAGE, AND UNHEALTHY GROUP OF 1,000 MEN

These actuarial tables and charts demonstrate the differences between the healthy, average, and the unhealthy groups. Clearly, the health implications of harmful lifestyle choices are substantial. Poor health choices exact a tremendous personal cost, increase medical expenses, and undermine the nation's health.

Harmful habits, such as tobacco, obesity, and inactivity, are epidemics threatening the good health of the entire nation. Some experts speculate that these epidemics may even be severe enough to reverse the recent improvements in life expectancy.

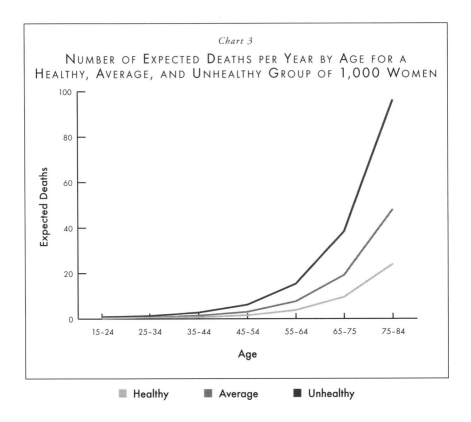

Chart 3

NUMBER OF EXPECTED DEATHS PER YEAR BY AGE FOR A
HEALTHY, AVERAGE, AND UNHEALTHY GROUP OF 1,000 WOMEN

▨ Healthy   ▨ Average   ■ Unhealthy

MEDICINE AND U.S. LIFE EXPECTANCY?

But, you say, Americans enjoy one of the highest standards of living on earth and spend the most on health care. Can't we buy our way to better health?

The short answer is "No."

Achieving the best health is not the same as possessing the most expensive medical care. In fact, the best health is the result of the very inexpensive preventive health choices this book promotes.

Want proof? Look at the next two sections on America's ranking among countries and the life expectancy of immigrants to America.

First, where do you think America ranks in life expectancy? In the top 5, top 10, top 20, top 50? Is American life expectancy closer to that of Japan or Cuba?

Take a look. America has nowhere near the best life expectancy. Surprised? America ranks 48th among all countries in life expectancy—*and our poor lifestyle choices account in large measure for our poor ranking.*

The numbers in table 7 are taken from the *World Fact Book* from the Central Intelligence Agency.[12] The table shows clearly that the health of the average American is not nearly as good as it should be. Would you expect our average life expectancy to be only slightly ahead of Cuba's? Well, that's where it is.

Table 7

COUNTRIES RANKED BY LIFE EXPECTANCY

(Data compiled by the U.S. Central Intelligence Agency, 2004 estimates)

Rank	Country	Life expectancy at birth (years)
1	Andorra	83.50
2	Macau	82.03
3	San Marino	81.53
4	Singapore	81.53
5	Hong Kong	81.39
6	Japan	81.04
7	Switzerland	80.31
8	Sweden	80.30
9	Australia	80.26
10	Iceland	80.18
11	Guernsey	80.17
12	Canada	79.96
13	Cayman Islands	79.81
14	Italy	79.54
15	Gibraltar	79.52
16	France	79.44
17	Monaco	79.42
18	Liechtenstein	79.40
19	Spain	79.37
20	Norway	79.25
21	Israel	79.17
22	Jersey	79.09
23	Faroe Islands	79.05
24	Aruba	78.98
25	Greece	78.94
26	Martinique	78.88
27	Austria	78.87

Table 7 continued

COUNTRIES RANKED BY LIFE EXPECTANCY

(Data compiled by the U.S. Central Intelligence Agency, 2004 estimates)

Rank	Country	Life expectancy at birth (years)
28	Virgin Islands	78.75
29	Malta	78.68
30	Netherlands	78.68
31	Luxembourg	78.58
32	Germany	78.54
33	Montserrat	78.53
34	New Zealand	78.49
35	Belgium	78.44
36	Saint Pierre and Miquelon	78.28
37	United Kingdom	78.27
38	Finland	78.24
39	Isle of Man	78.16
40	Guam	78.12
41	Jordan	78.06
42	Guadeloupe	77.71
43	Bermuda	77.60
44	Saint Helena	77.57
45	Puerto Rico	77.49
46	Cyprus	77.46
47	Denmark	77.44
48	United States	77.43
49	Ireland	77.36
50	Portugal	77.35
51	Albania	77.06
52	Taiwan	77.06
53	Cuba	76.90

MORE PROOF

Are you astonished that American life expectancy ranks so poorly? Wait until you read this next statistic. California studied its population and found that immigrants to this country live about three years longer than their California-born relatives despite getting less health care. The working hypothesis is that the immigrants have not yet adopted America's bad health habits. Instead, immigrants continue their traditional diets and exercise habits. Look at some details from the study:[13]

◆ Immigrants in California live, on average, 81.5 years, compared to 77.4 years for their U.S.-born relatives.

◆ All of the Asian subgroups, except Laotians and Cambodians, lived longer than California's state average.

◆ Asian Indians recorded the highest life expectancy among the 19 ethnic groups studied, which included white, black, Mexican, Cuban, Japanese, Chinese, Filipino, and Vietnamese[14]: 84.3 years—followed by Vietnamese (83.8 years), Chinese (83.7 years), and Koreans (83.2 years).

The immigrants fared better, even though they did not see a physician or get as much medical care as their U.S.-born counterparts. Quite simply, immigrants did not assimilate our fast-food culture or adopt our drive-everywhere mentality. Overall, they were thinner and did not smoke as much. The central messages?

1. There is more to be gained from low-tech preventive medicine than from our high-tech, expensive health care. Modern medicine can make us well, but it cannot keep us healthy. Good health in the 21st century will be determined more by diet and exercise than stomach staples and coronary stents.

2. We have the option to choose our health. We can choose good health with minimal disease and an active long life. Our lifestyle and health choices do matter. A lot.

PREVENTION IS THE ONLY WAY TO GO

Healthy choices translate directly to less disease, less disability, more activity, and longer life. The opposite is also true. Poor health choices will translate into more disease, costly health care, more time spent disabled or dependent upon others, and earlier death. There's just no way around it.

High-tech modern medicine can't treat smoking or a sedentary lifestyle or obesity. There are no magic pills that will provide all of the health requirements we need, no potions, no technology to keep us well or stop the biological processes our bad habits have set in motion. Choosing good health options many times a day is our responsibility. We cannot simply hope that we will live long enough for medical science to discover how to undo what we have done to ourselves.

Chapter 4

DON'T LET YOUR LIFE
GO UP IN SMOKE

To put it quite simply, healthy people don't smoke—not cigarettes, pipes, or cigars. So damaging are the effects of smoking that it's not possible to smoke and consider yourself healthy at the same time. You can eat wisely, exercise daily, control your blood pressure, and lower your cholesterol; but if you still smoke, all of those good habits only make you a healthier smoker. That's because using tobacco causes premature illness, prolonged disability, and death. There's no way around it. Tobacco use is the largest cause of premature death in America today.

The good news is that even after years of smoking, your body starts to recover immediately when you quit. The recovery process is both remarkable and rapid. Even if you are a smoker with heart disease, you can be reassured that your heart will heal more quickly if you stop smoking.

WHAT HAPPENS WHEN YOU CHOOSE TO QUIT?

When you choose to quit smoking, the harmful effects of that last smoke begin to wane. The short-term harmful impact of tobacco lessens. And in the long term, your body begins to heal itself.

Here's what the American Cancer Society says will happen when you quit smoking.[15]

- *Within hours* of your last smoke, your blood vessels relax and blood flows more normally. Your blood pressure begins to fall, moving toward the normal range. The temperature in your hands and feet rises. Your blood becomes more fluid, less sticky. Your risk of a heart attack decreases.

- *Within days,* your sense of taste and smell improves. You also smell better to those around you.

- *Within weeks,* your cough and your morning headache begin to clear.

- *Within 3 months,* your lung function improves by 30%.

- *Within 1 year,* you have lowered your risk of heart disease by half, compared to when you used to smoke.

- *Within 5 years,* your risk of a stroke equals that of a non-smoker.

- *Within 10 years,* your risk of lung cancer is now about half that of a smoker.

- *Within 15 years,* your risk of heart disease is the same as that of a person who never smoked.

You smoked for years; it will take years for your body to get better.

HELENA, MONTANA: A CASE IN POINT

Helena, Montana, a town of 65,000, has one hospital. For years, this hospital averaged seven heart attacks a month. In 2002, the city council banned smoking in public places, workplaces, bars, and restaurants. Almost immediately, the heart-attack rate dropped by 40% to an average of four heart attacks per month. Unfortunately, when the council repealed the smoking ban six months later, heart attacks rose again to six per month.[16] What is so amazing about Helena's story is how quickly the health of the whole community improved with the smoking ban.

THE COSTS OF SMOKING

Smoking is expensive in many ways. Smoking

◆ is the leading cause of premature disability and death,

◆ increases the number of times you will be ill,

◆ drives up the cost of your medical care and life insurance premiums.

The cumulative health costs of 40 million American smokers add up to some very large numbers. Each pack of cigarettes translates into $3.50 in additional medical care. Approximately 8% of all personal health care costs in America are related to smoking.[17] Each year, smoking costs the U.S. economy $100 to $150 billion in health-care costs and lost productivity.[18]

SMOKING AND FAMILIES

Smoking may be a personal choice, but there are family and societal costs associated with your choice to smoke. For example, maternal smoking causes premature births, small babies, and childhood asthma. At least half of all smoking mothers continue to smoke during their pregnancy, despite their best intentions to quit.

Many people start smoking when they are teens. Currently, around 20% of all high schoolers are considered smokers. Furthermore, the health risks of smoking begin even during these teenage years. Note: If your teen has not smoked by age 19, he or she is highly unlikely to ever pick up the habit.

Dr. Bob says:

◆ *Smoking or obesity or inactivity or a poor diet cancels the health protection of youth.*

Smoking at home exposes your family and friends to second-hand smoke. Think of tobacco smoke as an environmental toxin which substantially increases asthma attacks and respiratory diseases in kids and is unequivocally associated with an increased risk of heart disease and cancer. The degree of the increase caused by second-hand smoke is hotly debated, but not the fact that environmental tobacco smoke is harmful. If you love your significant other and your kids, don't smoke inside the car or the house.

SMOKING IS LETHAL

For decades, we've known that smoking is lethal. In the 1970s, the Surgeon General's report said that smoking a pack of cigarettes a day took seven years off your life. Since then, the average life expectancy of nonsmokers has grown by five years. The life expectancy of smokers has not kept pace. The gap between the life expectancy of smokers and nonsmokers may now be as much as 10 years, particularly when compared to the people who make good health choices.

- ◆ One in four smokers will develop a smoking-related disease or die before age 60.

- ◆ Smoking is responsible for 450,000 premature deaths per year.

- ◆ Smoking causes 90% of all lung cancer and much of cancer of the mouth, throat, and esophagus. If you and I were in charge, we could reduce all cancer deaths by 30% within a single generation by prohibiting smoking.

- ◆ Smoking causes at least 20% of all premature heart disease and peripheral vascular disease.

Figure 4, based on a British study of physicians who smoked, clearly shows the relationship between smoking and death.[19] Take a moment to look at the lines on the chart. They send a crystal clear message. At age 70, nearly 80% of the people who don't smoke are alive while only 50% of those who smoked more than 25 cigarettes per day are alive. At age 85, 33% of the nonsmokers are still going strong—but a mere 8% of the smokers are still alive, and I doubt they are going strong.

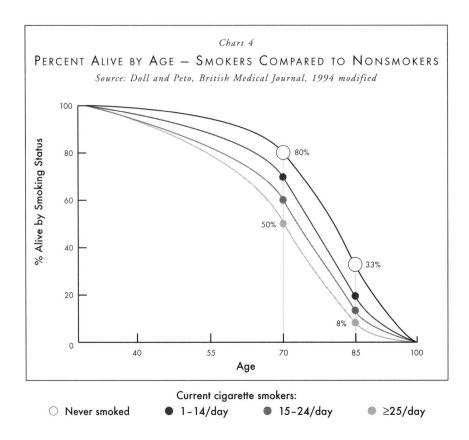

Chart 4

PERCENT ALIVE BY AGE — SMOKERS COMPARED TO NONSMOKERS

Source: Doll and Peto, British Medical Journal, 1994 modified

Current cigarette smokers:

○ Never smoked   ● 1–14/day   ● 15–24/day   ● ≥25/day

HOW FEW CIGARETTES, HOW MUCH DAMAGE?

Now, you might say you don't smoke "that much." So what happens if you smoke "just a little" or have an "occasional" cigarette?

Smoking even one cigarette can cause the kind of biochemical changes that lead to heart disease. In a recent study, a group of men smoked one—just one—cigarette. The researchers found that one cigarette lowered antioxidants in the blood stream, increased platelet stickiness, raised blood pressure, and stopped blood vessels from releasing nitric oxide, which normally works to keep blood vessels relaxed and open.[20] What does all of this mean?

These are the kind of changes that start to damage the inner lining of artery walls. We know the end result of this damage as atherosclerosis or hardening of the arteries. One cigarette makes your blood sticky and it starts to clot along the cholesterol-roughened artery walls, turning into the disease we call a heart attack. If one cigarette can do that much damage, imagine what a pack a day for 40 years does!

Smoking also causes emphysema, chronic bronchitis, impotence, ulcer disease, and vision loss. It increases bone loss and hastens osteoporosis. And for those who worry about the cosmetic dimension, smoking gives you yellow teeth, bad breath, and premature wrinkles.

MONEY SAVED BY QUITTING

Not only does smoking kill us prematurely, it does so at a tremendous cost. How much money could the country save if more people kicked the habit? If only 1% of the smokers stopped smoking, Americans would have almost 1,000 fewer heart attacks and 500 fewer strokes, saving approximately $44 million of medical costs in the first year alone.[21]

But this savings continues and multiplies because the effect of quitting becomes greater over time. If this 1% of the population continued to be smoke-free for seven years, the nation would reap the benefits of an estimated 63,840 fewer hospitalizations for heart attacks and 34,366 fewer hospitalizations for strokes. What does that mean in dollars? A savings of about $3.2 billion.[22]

Quitting

I know that if you're a smoker you have heard such sobering facts and figures before, but they underscore the need for making conscious, well-informed choices.

No one ever said quitting was easy. Yet here's the reality: you make a health choice every time you light up. Every time you light up, a great many awful things happen inside you. Many smokers would like to quit and have already tried several times. Most people try to quit seven times before they succeed. To help avoid the pitfalls of such a failure rate and increase your chances of succeeding, you will need a strategy, a support group, and nicotine withdrawal medication. But know this: you can quit.

Since tobacco is so powerfully addictive, quitting takes a very clear and concrete plan. It's something you should set down in writing. Think of it as a written plan, one that may help save your life as well as your money. How much money? By quitting, you can save yourself hundreds to thousands of dollars per year. That's the cost of a pack of cigarettes per day.

In your plan, you should write down your goal and the steps you will take to achieve the goal. You should also include a list of stumbling blocks that you are anticipating, what specific actions you will take to overcome them, and any outside help you'll need. Since you're making a plan, a sort of contract with yourself, you'll need to formalize the details. Here are some pointers.

1. Write a contract.

At the top of a piece of paper, write something like, "My Personal Plan to Quit Smoking." Decide when you want to quit, and commit to the date in a statement: "I will quit smoking on June 18, 2005, and I will not smoke again. Ever."

2. Add up the savings.

Total the money you spend on cigarettes per week. Now think of that as cash money in your pocket. Think of that much money after a year of not smoking. This is your monetary reward. Write down how you are going to save it or spend it. Then write down how good that will make you feel.

3. Focus on benefits.

The extra money you save is only one bonus, so you should also list other benefits of quitting. Here are a few to get you started.

◆ You'll have sweeter breath and whiter teeth.

◆ The smell of smoke won't cling to your clothes.

◆ No more little burn holes in clothing or upholstery. No more burn marks on the furniture.

◆ You'll be acting as a strong role model for your children and family as they watch you stick to your resolution.

◆ At work, you won't have to spend your break time outside in the rain, the cold, or the snow smoking with the others who can't wait to get out there.

◆ You will breathe more easily day by day.

◆ Your health will be better.

◆ Your life and health insurance premiums will be lower.

4. Review the benefits periodically.

Your list of benefits becomes really important about a month after you have quit. When you still want a cigarette, you will look at your list to review all the good reasons you are doing this. Whenever your cravings arise, review these benefits to help you stay focused. In fact, you may have to return to this document many times to bolster your determination. Half of all smokers try to quit every year. Unfortunately, kicking the habit for more than a year is very difficult. Having something that helps remind you of your goal and the good that will come of it will help strengthen your resolve.

5. Anticipate hurdles.

Identify obstacles to quitting, and record specific ways to overcome them. Help yourself by being proactive. To do this, think about situations when you enjoy smoking and how you can alter or avoid those situations to try to lessen your craving. For example, if you smoke at breakfast, go somewhere else for breakfast. If your family smokes, get them to quit with you, so you aren't tantalized by the smell of smoke.

6. Use nicotine replacement therapy.

Nicotine replacement therapy offers real help because these medications double your chance of succeeding. Look into the various nicotine replacement methods—gum, patch, nasal spray, or inhaler—to see which is best for you. Learn when and how to use the various forms because each one has a different nicotine delivery pattern and release time. For example, nicotine in gum is released 20–30 minutes after you start to chew. The medication is absorbed through your cheek, so the gum should be chewed and then parked next to the cheek for a minute.

Talk to your physician on how best to use the nicotine replacement. Write down how and when you will take your nicotine substitute so you minimize mistakes. For example, if you know you are going to crave a cigarette after your morning cup of coffee, then chew the gum before you have the coffee. Note: you cannot drink coffee (or any liquid) while chewing the gum because it dilutes the nicotine.

7. Try a medication to reduce cravings.

A non-nicotine prescription drug called Bupropion has been approved by the FDA as a medication that reduces nicotine cravings. Studies have shown that this medication increases the success rate among people who are trying to quit.

8. Develop tactics.

List anything you will call on for support, both short- and long-term. Write down what you will do when the urge to smoke hits. The urge will occur and it will pass. Will you take a walk, leave the table, chew some gum? This list can change and grow as you learn techniques that work best. But you must have a plan in place to help get past the urge to start again.

9. Broadcast the plan.

Now the scary part. Start telling your family, friends, and coworkers that you plan to quit. By voicing this commitment to others, you reinforce your commitment to yourself. You will find that this circle of people will encourage and support you in your efforts.

10. Keep thinking positively.

And then the even scarier part comes the moment after you've stubbed out your last cigarette or cigar or emptied your last pipe.

Tell yourself that you can do this. Your urges to smoke will pass and eventually lessen. Make "I can do this" into a mantra that you can repeat to affirm your goal.

11. Don't worry about extra pounds.

Keep this in mind: the few pounds you may gain are of little consequence compared to the health risks of smoking. Your weight has to double to equal the risk of smoking.

12. Be proud: just continue to not smoke.

It will be difficult, but you will be proud of yourself because it is difficult. Those within the circle of your support will be proud of you, too. While they may never have experienced the cravings themselves, they know that quitting is not easy. You need to keep telling yourself that quitting is essential to the rest of your life. Quitting will give you the rest of your life.

Chapter 5

THE FOUNTAIN OF YOUTH
IS A GLASS OF WATER
A MILE AWAY

ACTIVITY AND EXERCISE, THE MOST
BENEFICIAL PRESCRIPTION

Physical activity may be the single best medical treatment to prevent or treat disease. Unfortunately, physical activity is almost never prescribed. The real shame is that physical fitness can be achieved so easily by so many and its health benefits are so great.

Physical fitness is not limited to a fitness center and workout regimen. Being physically fit means you have at least a moderate level of cardiovascular fitness, strength, and flexibility. Being physically fit means you can do the physical activities you love for a long time.

Left to our own devices, very few of us get enough exercise. If you say you have no time to exercise, you are not alone. At today's hectic pace, very few people can find the time. And we are all confused about how much of what kind of exercise is enough. The result? Today Americans get less exercise than anytime in history and maybe less than anywhere else in the world.

Why is fitness important? What are the differences between fit and unfit people? So how much exercise is enough to be physically fit? "Official" recommendations have ranged from the hard-driving "no pain-no gain" school to the more laid-back "vacuuming counts as exercise" proponents. Some experts have said you must run every day, the farther the better. Others have said you must exercise one hour every day. Still others have said that you can exercise in 10-minute sessions a couple of times a day. No wonder you throw up your hands in confusion and dismay. It is easier to watch another hour of television than figure this out.

But you can't give up. Being active and fit is very important to your good health. In this chapter I'll explain how to benefit from activity and exercise. You will learn why fitness matters to your health, and what happens if you are inactive. Then you will learn what moderate exercise means and how to meet this target.

Dr. Bob promises:

◆ *You can get into much better physical shape without once going to the gym, and there's no need to buy new spandex workout clothes.*

◆ *You can start to be active more easily than you think, and you'll reap health benefits sooner than you think.*

As always when traveling this path to better health, I will ask you to make an informed choice. In this case, the choice is as simple as "Do you really want to watch this *Seinfeld* rerun for the fourth time, or do you want to reduce your risk of heart disease, cancer, and diabetes by taking a 30-minute walk?" The logic is obvious. It's the *doing* that we have to focus on. Let's see just how much you already do.

ARE YOU PHYSICALLY FIT?

Very few people really know whether they are fit. The only way to know is to perform some simple fitness testing on yourself. Go to the YMCA web site (http://www.exrx.net/Testing/YMCATesting.html) and you can find great tests to gauge your fitness. I recommend the one-mile-walk test for cardiovascular fitness, the push-up, sit-up tests, and the sit-and-reach flexibility tests. All of these will give you instructions for taking aerobic, strength, and stretch tests. The results are calculated, and your score is reported according to your age and gender. You should take these physical tests for the same reasons that you should know your cholesterol and your bank balance. They are a prediction of things to come and the only way to measure progress toward your goal.

Until you can log onto the YMCA fitness tests, take the brief quiz below. While the chart may not be scientific, it will tell you what you need to know.

Self-assessment 1. Test your fitness HOW MUCH EXERCISE DO YOU GET? CHECK THE BOXES THAT APPLY TO SEE WHERE YOU STAND.				
How would you describe yourself?	Inactive	Maybe not sedentary, but certainly not active	Pretty active	Very active
Do you exercise?	I do not and have no plans to start.	My intentions are good, but my follow-through is weak.	I get 30 minutes of brisk walking on most days, but I exercise inconsistently.	I get more than 30 minutes of play, activity, or exercise 4 or more days a week. I've done this for years.
Can you walk a mile?	That's what the internal combustion engine is for.	It has been a long time since I walked a mile, but I am pretty certain I can do it.	I usually walk more than 3 miles an hour.	I often take a long walk or run, moving at more than 4 miles an hour.
How much television do you watch?	My Lazy Boy is the best seat in the house. I use it every night.	I watch a couple of hours per day and even more on the weekend.	I watch an hour or two at a time, but not every day.	I am way too busy to watch television.
If you bend forward, which can you touch?	My knees	My ankles	My toes	Past my toes
% of U.S. population that falls into the category (approximate)	40%	30%	20%	10%

WHICH FITNESS GROUP ARE YOU IN?

The inactive. So where do you stand? Or do you prefer to sit?
Federal studies on exercise show that 70% of Americans are not

active (see chart 5). More than half of this 70% is *totally* sedentary, and the other half gets so little exercise that it doesn't count. If you belong to this group and have no scheduled fitness activities and do not get regular physical activity, you should think of yourself as facing a potential health risk.

Before you recoil at this dire prediction and begin to say that your days are filled with "some" activity, let's check the quality of that activity. You could think you are exercising, but you actually may fall into the group that is not active enough for their effort to improve their health. For example, you may say that you "enjoy walking," but to you, walking is really strolling at about two miles an hour, way too slow to count as exercise.

And walking around at work doesn't count either. You drive to work, walk from the parking lot to the office, walk to the water cooler, walk to the copy machine, walk to lunch, to the copier again, to the printer, to the car, and then home again. At the end of the day, you have maybe walked a mile and a half total and you're exhausted. Or perhaps you play golf regularly, but you always ride in the cart. If you're tired at the end of the day, your fatigue is far more likely the result of your physical weakness than your "workout."

Lack of activity only worsens as we age. A full three-quarters of the population over age 75 exercise not at all or so little that it does not count.

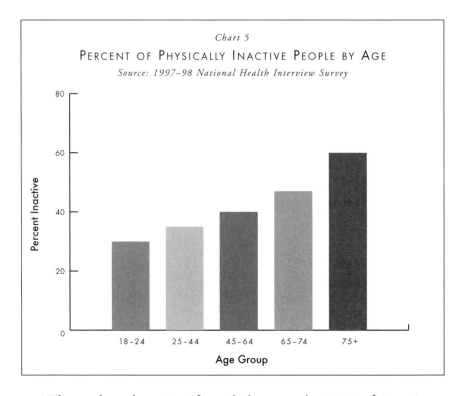

Chart 5

PERCENT OF PHYSICALLY INACTIVE PEOPLE BY AGE

Source: 1997–98 National Health Interview Survey

The moderately active. If you belong to the 20% of Americans who get moderate daily exercise and have done so for most of their life, you are reducing your health risks and promoting your health. How much activity is moderate? At least 30 minutes a day of physical activity or exercise four or more days a week. It does not matter what the activity or exercise is. You can walk briskly at lunch time, ride a stationary bike in the evening, do calisthenics or aerobics, play tennis, or jog. You can swim, ride a bike, take a hike, play Frisbee, or dance the tango.

If you belong in this group, chances are you've been active for most of your adult life. You are likely to do both your regular 30 minutes of exercise and to be more active in everything you do. You walk faster in the grocery store, garden more actively, or choose an active vacation. You play sports rather than just watch them. Because of this activity, you will develop fewer diseases or, if you get ill, typically you'll get ill later in life and recover faster. Your life will be longer and substantially more active.

A case in point: In the Nurses' Health Study, which traced 72,000 nurses, the group who walked 2.5 hours per week at more than 3 mph (their definition of moderate activity), showed 30% less coronary heart disease and stroke, compared to the inactive nurses.[23]

The very active. And then there are the 10% of Americans who exercise vigorously, seven days a week. This group enjoys the good feeling that comes with being fit and being able to do whatever they want. Their physical activities range from daily brisk walking to long-distance bicycling to yoga. Age doesn't make any difference to them.

The emeritus chair of this high-fitness club is Jack LaLanne, who at age 89 is as fit as many 30-year-olds. LaLanne has exercised fanatically his entire adult life, clearly demonstrating the benefits of his health program as he aged. When LaLanne was 45, he did 1,000 push-ups and 1,000 chin-ups in less than 90 minutes. At age 70, he swam a mile and a half while towing 70 boats. At age 89, he still works out for two hours every morning in his gym and swimming pool. He still travels the country, speaking and selling his products.

THE COST OF BEING INACTIVE

Most Americans fall into the inactive/sedentary category and, as a result, face a significant risk of chronic disease, impaired health, disability, and premature death because of their inactivity. However, as you will see, the good news is that this group can almost immediately gain health benefits by starting a moderate exercise program. If you belong to this group, you can regain strength as well as muscle tone and achieve fitness. You are never too out of shape or too old to start an exercise plan that will give you real health benefits.

"You don't get old from doing too much. You get old from doing too little."

— Jack LaLanne

Here's a hard-to-believe fact: if you are an inactive or sedentary person, your health risk is the same as a person who smokes a pack of cigarettes every day. That's how significant your health risks are if you are inactive. Dr. Manu Chakravarthy and Dr. Frank Booth, authors of the book *Exercise*, refer to the disease of being inactive as the "sedentary death syndrome."

Inactive people share these higher risks with smokers: a greater incidence of chronic diseases like heart disease and diabetes which will happen sooner and cause both longer periods of disability and premature death. Both groups tend to die 7 to 10 years before active people or nonsmokers. Take a look at some more numbers:

◆ In 1996, the Surgeon General added *sedentary lifestyle* to the list of factors that cause heart disease: 200,000 deaths annually can be attributed to a lack of exercise.

◆ The World Health Organization (WHO) named a sedentary lifestyle as one of the 10 leading causes of death and disability in the world. WHO noted that physical inactivity increases all the conditions that cause death, and doubles the risk of cardiovascular disease, type 2 diabetes, and obesity.

◆ A sedentary lifestyle also increases the incidence of colon and breast cancer, high blood pressure, lipid (cholesterol) disorders, osteoporosis, and arthritis, as well as depression and anxiety.

Astonishing, isn't it? And scary.

But the story need not be scary. Remember I said that the incredibly good news is that it is never too late to begin getting in better shape. An inactive 55-year-old can still become stronger, lose weight, and prevent heart disease and diabetes. A sedentary 65-year-old can start a physical fitness program and get into good enough shape to enter the Senior Olympics. A physically fit 70-year-old can be in better shape than an inactive 25-year-old. Even a frail 90-year-old can start a weight-lifting program to reduce the possibility of falling and breaking a bone.

Who Are the Inactive?

Clearly, being inactive is not healthy, yet the *inactive* group makes up 70% of the nation's population. Who are they? The answers will surprise you. They are people of all ages, from children to the elderly. In these days of computer games and television, children often can be as sedentary as the elderly. Inactive people cross all classification lines. They belong to all educational and socioeconomic classes; they are rich and poor, male and female. Some people make a conscious decision to avoid all forms of exercise and activity. Others simply slide into the inactive ranks because their work life robs them of the time they could use to be active. For still others, unwinding in front of the television is a stronger lure than moving around.

If you ask young parents why they don't exercise, they will all tell you, "I can't find the time." If you ask parents of teenagers why they don't exercise, they will all tell you, "I can't find the time." The same is true of empty nesters and retirees. No one, it seems, can "find the time." However, if they don't start to exercise, soon their excuses will change. Then people will tell you, "I don't exercise because my knees hurt too much" or "I get too out of breath" or "I am too weak."

CAN THESE LIVES BE SAVED?

Larry drives 60 minutes to work five mornings a week. His work is classic American corporate, circa the first decade of the 21st century. Larry sits in a cubicle, working on a keyboard eight hours a day. His daily exercise is limited to walking 45 feet to the printer and back. He drives to lunch. At the end of the day, he spends another 60 minutes driving home. Larry will tell you that he is active around the house and yard. In reality, he sits on a riding lawn mower, and when on the golf course, he zips around on a golf cart. He water-skis a couple of times a year but much prefers to drive the boat while his wife and teenage kids ski. Mainly, he saves his free time for watching weekend sports on television.

Marcie is an extremely successful lawyer. She works hard for the good money she earns. She works 60 hours a week and sometimes more. To get some exercise, she belongs to an athletic club where she pays for classes in advance so she can attend whenever her time permits. She has made it to 17 classes in four years, but who is counting? Marcie tried a personal trainer, but she talked to a client on her cell phone the whole time she was supposed to be lifting weights. Oddly enough, her PDA doesn't seem to accept "fitness time" on its calendar. Marcie thinks that she must be getting enough exercise because every night when she gets home, she's worn out. She also has trouble with her weight and tries very hard to watch what she eats. But when she works this hard, it is difficult to expend the energy watching her diet. Best just to grab what she can as quickly as she can for the family. No time, not enough time.

Both Larry and Marcie are classic inactive Americans. The signs on their life path say, "Getting Weaker," "Losing Fitness," and "Gaining Weight." What's really happening to their bodies because of their inactivity? They are losing muscle and strength. They are less flexible. Their heart pumps less well, their muscles use oxygen less well, and even their internal biochemistry is changing. Their cholesterol values are out of whack, they cannot handle blood sugar efficiently. Their inactivity is leading them down the path that leads to increased risks and premature disease.

The really incredible news is that both Larry and Marcie can begin to get in better physical shape and reverse their ill health. But first, they have to learn why being active and fit makes a difference. Then they have to decide what they are going to do about it—when are they going to "find the time" to do it? Let's see if we can help them get more fit.

Being Inactive—a Closer Look

So what happens while an inactive person sits? Why is inactivity so dangerous and deadly? And if being inactive is so dangerous, why haven't you noticed problems already?

Look at it this way. We all know that left alone, things tend to fall apart. Iron rusts, water evaporates, and weeds grow in gardens. What's more, these are all gradual processes that advance over time. Our bodies are not much different.

Imagine that you are a 30-year-old inactive person. Every year after age 30, you will lose one-half pound of muscle. Between ages 30 and 60, despite no weight gain, you will turn 15 pounds of muscle into 15 pounds of fat. Said differently, you will lose between a quarter and half of your muscle mass between age 30 and age 65—unless you exercise.

This is how bodies work. During childhood, adolescence, and on into your 20s, your body builds muscle—it's biologically priming itself for reproduction and caring for young, which generally occurs in the third decade of life. Somewhere between age 20 and 30, all of your biological processes peak. You can run the fastest, play the longest, and work the hardest. Your bones have the most calcium. You can party almost all night.

After age 30—without some sort of active intervention, such as regular exercise—the natural law of entropy takes over. This law says that when things are left to themselves, including our bodies, they naturally start to fall apart. Don't dwell on this idea too long. Just recognize that muscles weaken and bones lose calcium unless you exercise. You become less flexible (have you?), and your balance slowly begins to decline. The changes are so subtle that we do not even notice them for several years.

This all happens very gradually. Although your strength may have started slipping many years ago, if you're like most people, men and women, you have enough muscle reserve to power your way through life until you hit age 60 or thereabouts. Then the losses in strength, balance, cardiovascular endurance, respiratory function, and flexibility reach the point where you notice them.

Turning muscle to fat is not a good trade. It starts you sliding down a slippery slope. As muscles weaken, you become less active, more sedentary, more out of shape. Because you are less active, you lose more muscle. The decline is subtle. For example, when you decide to start an exercise program or tackle the annual autumn yard cleanup, you find yourself weaker than the previous autumn. Unfortunately, when this happens, many people draw the wrong conclusion: they assume that they are old and stiff, and therefore, they should do even less activity in the future. Wrong. That stiffness is a sign you should be doing more.

And keep this in mind about fat. Fat is less metabolically active than muscle, meaning it burns fewer calories even at rest. When your muscle turns into fat, that additional 15 pounds of fat burns fewer calories than muscle. *Therefore, even if you eat exactly the same number of calories as you did at age 30, you will gain weight.* Your body has lost muscle and added extra weight—soon you are struggling to walk the golf course. What's more, because you're heavier, your sluggish body finds being active more difficult than it used to be. You have less incentive than ever to begin to exercise. And the decline begins to accelerate. Exercise and physical activity are the only ways to reverse the decline.

As a result, a 60-year-old marathoner is more fit than a 40-year-old couch potato. It is entirely possible for a 60-year-old of even modest physical condition to get into marathon shape. He will not run as fast as an in-shape 30-year-old, but our senior athlete will run a whole lot faster than his friends.

How Did We Become So Inactive?

The American way of life, our countless number of laborsaving devices, promotes inactivity. Think about it. Opening the garage door used to mean getting out of the car and lifting the door up. Garage door openers did not exist 50 years ago. Today, we push a button and drive away. Today we ride escalators instead of walking up stairs. We stand on moving sidewalks in airports. Our vacuum cleaners are self-propelled, and our car windows slide up and down at the push of a button. We even rely on automatic can openers (as though cranking open a can of peaches is an effort). Our CDs change themselves. We don't even leave our loungers to change a channel. Remotes are everywhere!

We have enthusiastically embraced these benefits, so much so that we no longer think that we can choose another way. And in some places we do not have a choice. Some golf courses require riding in golf carts and do not permit walking. In most suburbs—the land of no sidewalks—it's nearly impossible to walk from the grocery store to the pharmacy, so we end up driving the half-mile instead of walking.

Every one of these laborsaving devices permits us to exercise less. Viewed from another perspective, laborsaving can mean exercise preventing. And when this lack of activity is forced on us, society has mandated—not just encouraged—our inactivity.

Try this little experiment. Do without the television remote for one night. Getting out of the typical lounge chair is not much different than doing half a sit-up and a deep-knee bend. Without the remote, every time you change the channel, you are doing a half sit-up and a deep-knee bend. Channel surfing without a remote quickly becomes a mini-workout for the average male. Guys, would you really change the channel every nine seconds if you had to get out of your chair each time?

Amid all the laborsaving gizmos, it takes a concerted effort for you to make physical activity an integral part of your life. Identify the gizmos in your life that enable inactivity. Every chance you can, start to trade the inactive laborsaving option for the option that requires more effort. These little bits of activity may not be exercise, but they require that your muscles work, which is a good thing. You can walk up the escalator as it moves instead of standing still, you can sell your riding mower and buy a push mower, walk to the theater instead of grabbing a cab, or beat the eggs by hand rather than with a mixer.

Dr. Bob says:

- ◆ *Choose the path of more resistance.*

THE BENEFITS OF GETTING IN BETTER SHAPE

Regardless of your current state of fitness or lack of fitness, you can get into better physical condition. Everyone—and I mean even the most sedentary, out-of-shape person—can improve their fitness. Here's the motivator: moving from a sedentary lifestyle to some activity produces tremendous health benefits and takes less effort than you might guess.

Let me clarify. Getting into better shape does not mean being buff. It does not mean developing 6-pack abs. Improved conditioning does not necessarily mean jogging three miles uphill, wearing spandex, or hiring a personal trainer. Starting physical activity means walking more and faster and farther. It means adding any form of activity to your daily routine that you like and will do. Just taking the first steps toward becoming more active means you will burn more calories, build muscle, and strengthen bones. You will feel better and grow stronger. Then, little by little, you will feel like increasing your activity even more.

Dozens of medical studies involving hundreds of thousands of people confirm the benefits of exercise. Getting more active and starting to get the recommended 30 minutes of moderate exercise a day will lower your:

- ◆ risk of heart disease

- ◆ total cholesterol and raise the good HDL cholesterol

- ◆ blood pressure

- ◆ weight and help you maintain a normal weight

- ◆ risk of type 2 diabetes

◆ risk of osteoporosis

◆ risk of falls and broken bones

If you are ill, physical activity will help you get better.

◆ If you have had a heart attack, exercise will lower your risk of a second one.

◆ If you have diabetes, exercise will help you control your blood sugars.

◆ If you are depressed or stressed, exercise will help you feel better.

Think about all these things as you turn off the television and set off for a 30-minute walk.

Inactive people have problems with daily living, such as carrying two bags of groceries, picking up a shirt from the floor, and bending over to tie their shoes. And none of this is going to get any easier as they get older. Getting into better shape means regaining the ability to walk without being short of breath, knowing you can go through the airport without asking for a ride in a cart, and being flexible enough to know you won't get hurt while working in the yard. You'll have more confidence on your feet—feel stronger, stand straighter and taller. It means stronger bones, firmer arms and legs, a flatter tummy. Golf becomes more enjoyable. Gardening is easier. Playing with grandchildren is more fun. Sex is more satisfying. Everything is better.

Let's check in with Larry and Marcie.

By now, Larry is now a physical wreck. He's clearly overweight. Ten hours of commuting every week has taken its toll—either that, or his cleaners keep shrinking his clothes. His now 10-year-old twins, Susie and Steven, love sports and want Dad to practice with them after work. But Larry can't. He is simply not physically fit enough to be able to play. Every time he hustles to get a baseball or kicks a soccer ball, he gets winded within a few minutes. Then he hurts for the next few days. He knows this isn't good.

Larry is only 47. He and his wife have one of those "now dear" dinner conversations because they are both very worried about the example that their inactivity is setting for the children. She sends him off to the Mayo Clinic for an executive physical.

Marcie continues to plow through her work and climb the corporate ladder. In fact, she is now part of senior leadership in a new company with a real chance to hit the big time—that is, until her traffic accident. While her injuries were not major, she was bounced around a bit and came away with lots of bruises and a nagging back pain that would not go away. Her physician sent her to physical therapy, where she was given an exercise regimen and forced to participate. Fortunately, she had a tough-love physical therapist. Actually, maybe more tough than love. Marcie's Palm Pilot now had to accept the fitness times.

And she did show up, and the physical therapist really

did make her exercise. Marcie noted to herself that it was easier to arrange a corporate buyout than to do that third set of weights and stretches. On the other hand, this fitness regimen did have its strong points. She liked what was happening with her body. Plus, it was not all bad to get some time away from the office. The question for Marcie was, as always, would she continue to exercise or would the sirens of business call her back to the office?

WHAT DOES SCIENCE SAY ABOUT FITNESS?

Scientific studies abundantly support the benefits of activity and exercise. Let's briefly look at just a few studies that emphasize how active lifestyles prevent disease and death.

1. Being active is healthy.

Dr. Ralph Paffenbarger of Stanford University recently studied 17,000 Harvard alumni who graduated between 1916 and 1950. He learned two important things. First, the group of men who were active had half the death rate of the inactive group.[24] Second, vigorous activity was better than moderate activity which, in turn, was better than no activity.[25] A lifetime of activity was more important than playing college athletics. Dr. Paffenbarger found that even college varsity sports offered no protection if the alum later became sedentary. Dr. Paffenbarger classified the Harvard alumni on reports of how much they walked, the number of stairs they climbed per day, and the amount of sports they actively played.

2. The health benefit of being active starts with relatively small amounts of exercise.

Dr. Amy Hakim studied 700 nonsmoking men of similar health habits as part of the Honolulu Heart Study. These men entered the study between 1980 and 1982 when they were between ages 45 and 68. At that time, they were asked how far they walked. Ten years later, the men were again asked how far they walked. There was a clear association between the distance walked and cancer, heart disease, and all causes of mortality. As the chart below shows, the risk of death for men who walked less than a mile a day was almost two times greater than for men who walked more than two miles a day.[26]

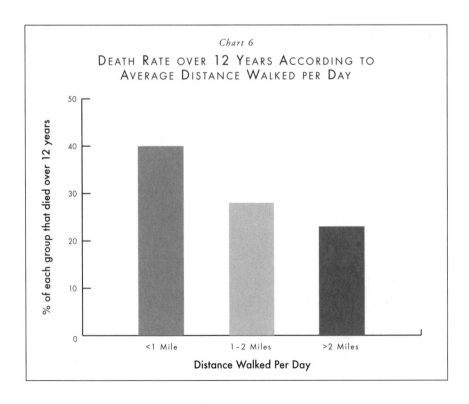

Chart 6

DEATH RATE OVER 12 YEARS ACCORDING TO AVERAGE DISTANCE WALKED PER DAY

3. Some vigorous exercise is beneficial, but more is better.

A Finnish study[27] of 16,000 male and female identical twins between 1977 and 1994 showed results very similar to the Honolulu Heart Study. In this study, people were divided into three groups: the sedentary, who had no leisure time activity; the occasional exercisers, who exercised some but less than six times a month; and the conditioned exercisers, who exercised more than six times a month at the equivalent of 30 minutes of jogging or vigorous walking per session.

Table 8 EVEN SMALL AMOUNTS OF REGULAR PHYSICAL EXERCISE ADD BENEFIT		
Group	Definition	Overall death rate
Inactive	No leisure time activity	12.0%
Occasional exercisers	Exercised some but less than 6 times a month	7.4%
Conditioned exercisers	Exercised more than 6 times a month at the equivalent of 30 minutes of jogging or vigorous walking	4.9%

4. Being active is beneficial even for people with other risk factors.

Dr. Steven Blair, a leading expert in the health benefits of exercise, studied 25,000 men and 7,000 women who went to the Cooper Clinic for executive physicals for 20 years. He divided the group in fifths based on their fitness measurements. He found the least physically fit 20% of the people had a 70% higher risk of death from cardiovascular disease than the most fit 20%. He wrote, "The protective effect of fitness held for smokers and non-smokers, those with and without elevated cholesterol levels or elevated blood pressure, and healthy and unhealthy persons."[28]

The graph below shows the huge health gain achieved simply by moving from the lowest group (the 20% who exercised the least) to the second group (the 20% who were somewhat active). The people in the lowest group were truly sedentary and did no physical activity. People entered the second-lowest group of fitness if they walked 30 minutes a day at a moderate pace.

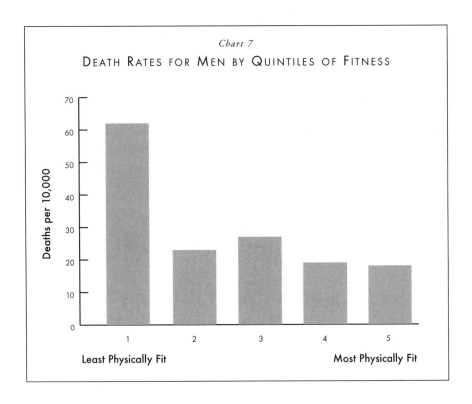

Chart 7
DEATH RATES FOR MEN BY QUINTILES OF FITNESS

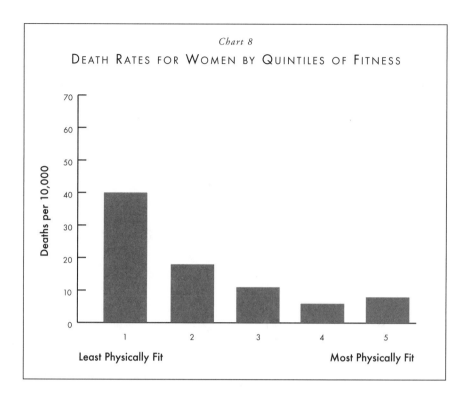

Chart 8

DEATH RATES FOR WOMEN BY QUINTILES OF FITNESS

5. *The inactive person who abandons the recliner for walking reaps greater benefits than the already active walker who trains for a marathon.*

A sedentary person gets a larger health benefit from starting to walk briskly 30 minutes a day than an average exerciser gets by becoming a marathoner (see charts 7 and 8 above). Notice the relative differences between fitness groups 1 and 2. Going from sedentary to some activity produces a much larger improvement than the difference between fitness group 4 and 5, with 5 being the marathoners.

6. Even if a person starts in the inactive group, he or she can get active and reap the health benefit.

In another study, Dr. Blair identified nearly 10,000 people who had at least two exams at the Cooper Clinic.[29] The researchers compared three groups: (1) those who were unfit on both exams, (2) those who started as unfit on the first exam but became fit by the second exam, and (3) those who were fit on both exams. Note the risk for premature death dropped almost 50% in the group that started to get active. This reinforces the idea that it does not matter where you start, only that you get going.

Table 9 AN UNFIT PERSON CAN IMPROVE HIS OR HER HEALTH BY STARTING TO GET ACTIVE	
Men	**Deaths per 10,000 person-years***
Unfit in both examinations	122
Improved from unfit to fit between first and second exams	68
Fit at both examinations	40

* Following 1,000 people for 10 years equals 10,000 person-years.

Dr. Bob says:

◆ *Starting an exercise program improves your health as much as stopping smoking.*

7. The benefit of exercise persists far into old age.

Perhaps the greatest benefit of activity is that it helps you avoid the decline that comes with normal aging. Dr. Lawrence Golding of the University of Nevada at Las Vegas compiled data on more than 1,000 adults in his exercise classes that meet three times a week. He agrees that the people who exercised two hours per week remain free of even minor disabilities for more than seven years longer than their nonexercising counterparts.[30] Dr. Golding is a coauthor of the National YMCA Physical Fitness Program. The exercises from his fitness classes are on his web site at http://www.unlv.edu/faculty/golding/. His program must work: he has 80-year-olds in his classes who have the strength, fitness, and flexibility of 30-year-olds.

A Summary of What the Studies Mean to You

The conclusion is clear. Being active is very important for good health. Every inactive or not-active-enough person can gain tremendous health benefits by starting to work his or her muscles.

1. Active people have less disease and live longer than inactive people.

2. The health benefits of activity start with as little as a brisk one-mile walk per day.

3. The more you exercise or are active, the better your health.

4. Being active is beneficial even if you have other risk factors.

5. A sedentary person gains more health benefits by becoming active than a fit person gains by becoming a marathoner.

6. Even if you are a couch potato, you can improve your health by starting to be more active.

7. Fit older people stay more active much longer.

Your new added activities can be minimal, but they should be progressive so that a year from now you are more active than today. At this point, it does not matter what the exercise is. You can walk or dance, play tennis, basketball, or badminton. Over time, many people switch their exercise of choice from aerobics to yoga to weight lifting to swimming to raquetball. Everyone should include daily exercise and activity as a lifelong habit. The point is that we need to be active for our entire lives. By choosing to be active, we choose greater strength, fulfillment, better health, and a longer life.

Dr. Bob promises:

◆ *Deciding to exercise may be the most important health decision you can ever make (assuming you do not smoke, of course).*

Let's check in with Larry.

When we last saw Larry, he was on his way to the Mayo Clinic for an executive physical. He went fearing that the doctors would find a dread disease. And while they did not find a dread disease, they did find a whole lot of troubling signs of impending heart disease and diabetes. Larry was obese with a body mass index of 36 (see chapter 6) and a waist measurement of 44 inches. A borderline diabetic, Larry's cholesterol levels were backward, with the bad LDL cholesterol too high and the good HDL cholesterol too low. His blood pressure was also borderline. Adding insult to injury, the Mayo physicians told him he was among the least fit 20% of the population. He learned that he was headed for serious medical trouble. The physician put Larry on an exercise program and sent him to a dietician. Fortunately, Larry listened. He walked away with a new goal: to become more physically fit, to start to eat right, and to lose some weight.

HOW MUCH EXERCISE IS ENOUGH?

If you are "inactive," you get little or no exercise, and you engage in only minimal physical activity. Typically, you watch several hours of television every day, and by the end of the day, you may feel tired. You are tired because you are so weak and out of shape that *any* activity, even grocery shopping or walking to a restaurant, can feel strenuous.

Question: How do you shake off this feeling of fatigue that comes with only mild exertion? Answer: Exercise.

All of the science studies in this chapter show that both men and women are much healthier if they get regular exercise. So the real question is, how much activity is enough?

At the outset, any exercise is better than none. But in order to be really beneficial, you have to exercise at least 30 minutes a day and the activity has to be at least as strenuous as walking briskly. The most commonly accepted recommendation is "30 minutes of moderate exercise on most days of the week."

You understand the 30-minute part, but what does "moderate exercise" mean?

Even at rest, you burn 70 to 100 calories per hour. People who study exercise refer to the energy you use at rest as one MET or the metabolic equivalent of the task. These experts then assign different activities as multiples of resting energy or MET multiples. Jogging, for example, is an eight-MET activity, so it burns eight times as much energy as resting.

"Moderate exercise" is defined as any activity that burns three to six times as much energy (calories) as you spend at rest. This can also be stated as a three- to six-MET activity. Moderate exercise then is roughly an activity that burns 300 calories per hour. So now you ask, how does 300 calories per hour translate into your everyday activities?

Table 10 organizes the information for you. It lists different activities and the energy used in the activity in METs and calories spent per hour. This chart will help you understand the relationship among different activities and their energy requirements.

You'll notice that Table 10 shows various activities arranged in order of increasing energy. Each activity shows the METs and the calories burned for an average-size person. Thus, by looking at the METs per hour, you can get an idea of the intensity of the activity. METs are included in the table because many exercise prescriptions and activities use METs.

Look at the table's Light Activity section. Clearly, the levels of activities listed are so close to resting that they cannot be termed exercise. Watching television burns only 100 calories per hour. Even rapid channel surfing won't get you to your exercise goal. Working in an office does not take much more energy, although it makes us more tired.

Table 10

COMMON ACTIVITIES ARRANGED IN ASCENDING ORDER OF CALORIES PER HOUR AND MET UNITS

Activity	Description	Calories per hour (for a 70-kg or 154-pound person)	METs
Light activity (50 to 250 kcal/hour) Does not count as exercise			
Resting	Resting	80	1.0
Watching television		100	1.0
Working in an office		110	1.5
Driving a car		110	1.5
Standing		140	2.0
Golf in a cart		150	2.0
Strolling	Walking 2.5 mph on level ground	150	2.5
Cycling slowly	5 mph	220	3.0
Moderate-intensity exercise (250 to 350 kcal/hour) The benefits of moderate exercise start at this level			
Walking	3 mph	300	3.3
Golf, walking the course		300	4.5
Cycling	10 mph	300	4.0
Walking briskly	3.5 mph	320	4.0
Walking very briskly	4 mph	350	4.5
Strenuous activity (more than 350 kcal/hour)			
Bicycling	10 mph	400–500	5.0–6.0
Tennis, singles		420–500	5.0–6.0
Dancing		400–600	5.0–8.0
Jogging or walking at 5 mph	5 mph	650	8.0
Jogging, moderate pace	6 mph	750	10.0
Running	10 mph	1,200	16.0

To learn more about the energy you expend while exercising, go to http://healthylife.umdnj.edu/archives/METsWork.htm or www.discoverfitness.com. Both sites give a fairly complete listing of exercises and activities, citing their MET units as well as calorie equivalents.

What Does This Mean for You?

Most of this discussion focuses on the energy requirements of different walking speeds because walking is the most popular exercise. Walking slowly at 2.5 mph on level ground burns only 150 calories per hour. But if you pick up the pace to a speed of between 3 and 3.5, or even 4 miles an hour—the pace you use when you're late for an appointment—you enter the moderate range. As soon as you get into jogging or its equivalent, you have passed into strenuous or vigorous exercise.

You can begin to meet the minimum requirement for *moderate exercise* by walking briskly for 30 minutes, four days a week. Here's an example. If your idea of a brisk walking speed is 3.5 mph, you will walk 1.75 miles on each of the four days. That is enough to meet the definition of "moderate exercise." If you weigh 154 pounds, you will burn 160 calories on your half-hour walk or 320 calories per hour walked. At the end of the week, you will have walked for two hours—a total of seven miles—and burned 640 calories.

Remember, the greatest benefit occurs for people who move from being sedentary or performing only light activity to a program that expends 700 calories per week. Think about it: you will burn 640 calories if you walk briskly for a total of two hours this week. Just about everyone ought to be able to manage this level of activity.

Unfortunately, burning 700 calories a week is not enough activity to lose weight. It's just enough activity to qualify you for the "moderately active" category. To start to lose weight and really reach the optimal level of fitness, you have to be closer to the 2,000 calories per week level. However, this still does not mean you have to go to the fitness center. Watch how easily we can all get to 2,000 calories per week.

Dr. Bob's prescription for exercise nirvana:

◆ *Start to walk everywhere as though you were late for an appointment. By picking up the pace like this, you will use more calories and make your body stronger. These little walks do not technically count as exercise, but they do make you stronger. It takes a minimum of 10 minutes of activity for your body to register a real health benefit.*

◆ *Now add three brisk 10-minute walks every day. To really get results, walk as if you are half a mile away from an appointment that starts in 3 minutes. Eat a 20-minute lunch and walk for 10 minutes. Park your car in the far corner of the parking lot and walk the extra steps to the office or store. Walk the long way home from school. These three 10-minute walks add up. Do 3 of these brisk 10 minute walks every day for a week and you have walked 3 1/2 hours. If you are an average-size person, you burned 320 calories per hour for 3 1/2 hours, or over 1,000 calories. Everyone pooh-poohs these 10-minute bits of exercise. Don't. They are a real key to fitness.*

◆ *Now every evening, turn off the television, go out the front door, turn left, walk for 15 minutes, turn around, and come home again. Do this four days a week and you add another*

640 calories. Take the 30-minute walk seven days a week, and now you are up to another 1,000 calories.

◆ *Add up all of these little times you chose to walk. Bingo! You are over 2,000 calories per week. You just walked your way to fitness nirvana.*

Once you get moving, you can expand your fitness activities to other areas: dancing, swimming, playing tennis, badminton, or any other physical activity of your choice.

A WARNING

Our ability to be physically active decreases naturally as we get older. For example, walking at a 4-MET pace may be light activity for a 30-year-old, but it's moderate activity for a 55-year-old and vigorous activity for a 75-year-old. Alternatively stated, moderate exercise for a 30-year-old means exercising at a 5-MET level; for a 50-year-old, moderate exercise is 4.5 METS; for a 65-year-old, moderate exercise is 4 METs; and for an 80-year-old, moderate exercise is closer to 2.5 METs. Keep your age in mind as you set your exercise goals.

FINDING THE TIME

Remember all of those groups earlier in the chapter who said that they didn't have the time to exercise? Here's how you do it. You rise from your couch and turn off the television. It's an even easier thing to do during the six months of the year known as rerun season. See, we are not talking about finding extra time in the day. We are talking about making an informed choice to better use the time we have.

Dr. Bob says:

◆ *We've yet to find a disease state where exercise isn't helpful.*

Walking for Weight Loss

Exercise and physical activity are always an integral part of any weight loss plan. Weight is "calories in" balanced against "calories out." To effectively lose weight, you must both decrease the calories you eat and increase the calories you burn in exercise. Exercise and physical fitness are the "calories out" part of the equation. Exercise helps you lose weight in a couple of ways:

1. Exercise and physical activity of any type burn calories.

2. Exercise builds muscle, and muscle burns more calories than fat, even at rest.

3. Exercise helps regulate blood sugar more efficiently.

When you walk to lose weight, you must increase at least two of these three: time, speed or distance. The people who promote the 10,000 steps program say that 10,000 steps are necessary for good cardiovascular health. But to lose weight you must walk 15,000 steps a day. See digiwalker.com for successful weight loss stories. These people all lost weight by limiting calories and by walking.

The calories you burn as you walk will vary depending on your speed, your weight, and the terrain. Tables 11 and 12 show the difference that your weight and walking speed will make in calories burned. A more precise calculator for merging individual weight, speed, and time walking can be found at www.preventdisease.com/healthtools.

Table 11

CALORIES BURNED BY WALKING FOR A 140-POUND PERSON

Minutes per mile	Miles per hour	Calories spent per mile	Calories spent per hour
30	2	87	174
20	3	96	288
15	4	82	328
12	5	105	525

Table 12

CALORIES BURNED BY WALKING FOR A 220-POUND PERSON

Minutes per mile	Miles per hour	Calories spent per mile	Calories spent per hour
30	2	125	250
20	3	188	396
15	4	231	462
12	5	376	752

Source: www.preventdisease.com/healthtools

SO WHAT ABOUT WEIGHT-TRAINING OR STRENGTH-BUILDING EXERCISES?

Now that you understand the powerful benefits of aerobic (cardiovascular) exercise, such as walking, we need to paint a picture of complete physical fitness.

Complete fitness requires all three types of exercises: aerobic, strength building, and stretching. Walking gives you cardiovascular or aerobic fitness. If you are a marathon walker, your legs and heart will be in great shape. But despite all your walking, your upper body strength could actually be quite poor, and your flexibility could be limited.

If you took the YMCA fitness tests mentioned in the early pages of this chapter, you'll recall that the tests measured cardiovascular fitness by a walking test, upper body/torso strength by counting push-ups and sit-ups, and flexibility by a forward stretch. Let's take a look at these other two areas of getting fit.

Weight-bearing exercise. Weight-bearing exercises strengthen muscles and bones. Strengthening exercises should be done twice a week. The goal is not to build big muscles. Rather, you are trying to strengthen your upper body so you are strong enough to be active.

Strengthening exercises are far more important than most of us acknowledge. Study after study demonstrates that people who lift weights or do other strengthening exercises gain far more than muscle. They gain strength, movement, and balance; their bodies feel and look younger; and they do more activities. Dr. Miriam Nelson, who wrote *Strong Women Stay Young,* notes that "after one year of strength training twice a week, women's bodies were fifteen to twenty years more youthful."[31]

You can choose whatever strength-building exercises you want. Here are just some exercises to choose from:

◆ push-ups and sit-ups

◆ preplanned and organized circuits at the fitness club

◆ yoga

◆ weight training

◆ old-fashioned calisthenics

Flexibility exercises. Your body is meant to move in many ways. A youngster can stretch, hop, throw a ball, twist sideways, and bend. How many of these can you do today?

Not only can't we move very well, but our upper body is frozen into a comma-like posture—hunched over in the mid-back and slouched forward. How did we get that way? Think of your day. You drive leaning forward, shoulders hunched. You sit at a keyboard, leaning forward, gazing at a monitor, shoulders hunched. You eat and talk on the phone using the same posture.

How often during a day do you arch backward or twist sideways? Can you raise your arms straight above your head? You should be able to. Can you throw a ball using the same motion you had 30 years ago? You should be able to. Can you stand on one foot for a minute? You should be able to.

Chances are you've forgotten how to do these common, everyday movements. The longer we do not stretch these joints and use these muscles, the stiffer and weaker we get. The more we neglect these actions and the weaker we get, the older we feel.

Remember: you can get back all the fitness and flexibility of your youth. Exercise and fitness, stretching and strength building can do wonders to rejuvenate your body. Once you have started to feel stronger and more physically confident, you will do more. Your actions become a self-fulfilling prophecy. Better health can be achieved after all. As Jack LaLanne says, "You don't get old from doing too much. You get old from doing too little." It is time for you to do more—to lift, to stretch, and to play.

GETTING STARTED

Most exercise plans quickly fail because our dreamed-of goals are unrealistic. An inactive and out-of-shape couch potato should not vault off the couch and sign up for next year's Olympics.

The worst mistake you can make is to go from inactive to hyperactive in a single weekend. This sudden push to fitness is doomed to fail. A sedentary person may be very weak, with very little cardiovascular reserve or strength. And any sort of exercise hurts. It's best to start slow and easy. The YMCA fitness site referenced above has excellent age-adjusted exercise programs to suit your current fitness score and age.

Your best path from inactivity to fitness is a planned, steady increase in walking time and speed, strengthening exercises, and stretching. This process of returning to fitness is slow, one that may take a year to achieve and a lifetime to maintain. You've got to remember that it took years of inactivity to get this out of shape. You should expect that it will take a few months, if not a year, to regain some fitness. A year is not a long time.

When people claim that they have no time for exercise, they think of exercise or physical fitness as driving to the gym (as if that makes any sense), changing clothes, exercising, showering, getting dressed, and driving home again. While that may be one way to get physically fit, it is certainly time-consuming. Little wonder then that no one has time to exercise.

You can actually find time for adding physical activity in five places in your busy day. In fact, you *must* start to add physical activity to your routines, but these activities don't take much time or interfere with your life.

1. First, sprinkle added activity throughout your workday.

Take the stairs instead of the elevator or escalator. Walk faster: pretend you're late and pick up the pace. The more you walk at this quicker pace, the sooner it will become natural for you, helping you take longer walks.

2. Exercise in 10-minute blocks.

Don't think you have any free time? Find three 10-minute blocks of time during your day. Here are some examples. How long does it take you to eat lunch? Maybe you want to walk as well as eat. If you eat out, how far away is the restaurant? If you are going to take 45 minutes for lunch, spend 10 minutes walking the long way to the restaurant, eat in 25 minutes, and then walk the route back. If you take the subway or bus to work, get off a stop too soon and walk the last several blocks. Have to wait for your child to finish soccer practice? Get out of the car and walk around for five minutes.

3. Find time by making different choices.

The average American watches four hours of television a day. How much of it is really that entertaining? In the time it takes you to watch a sitcom, you can walk a mile and a half, maybe two at a moderate pace. This walk may lower your risk of heart disease by 50%, help you lose weight, control your diabetes, increase bone strength, improve arthritis, and maybe lower the risk of some cancers. Maybe that reality show isn't so important after all.

4. Put these strategies together.

Soon you have the start of a real exercise program. Walk at least a few flights of stairs. Walk everywhere more quickly. Sneak in three 10-minute walks a day. Add a 30-minute walk every evening. When all is said and done, this totals an hour of brisk walking a day, and suddenly you're moving 20–30 miles a week. You'll burn 100–150 calories per mile, so these 20–30 miles will total 2,000 to 4,500 calories per week, depending on your walking speed and weight.

You will notice that your body is changing for the better. You'll start to lose weight. Your appetite may change as you begin to look for healthier foods to match your new activity level and new body. All of these factors carry you along the path to a much healthier you.

5. Lift weights and stretch.

As you start to feel more physically fit and more confident in your strength, you should add weight-bearing exercises and stretching exercises. There are dozens of programs, books, and videos to help you. Just remember that you do not want to burn out or hurt yourself. This is a path you'd like to travel for the rest of your life.

Think of exercise as a medical prescription from Dr. Bob: exercise 30 minutes a day. If your blood pressure were high, I might prescribe a medication and tell you change your diet. As you followed the prescribed treatment, your blood pressure would come down. How would you know? You would measure your blood pressure. If you stopped the treatment, your blood pressure would go back up. Walking for fitness is the same. You should be able to measure your progress by the ease and speed with which you walk. Over time, both will get better. You will continue to stay fit. Remember this: Can't jog? No big deal. Beginning a walking program at any age and continuing it for the next 55 years is far better than jogging for two years, hating it, and then quitting.

So to wrap up, the best exercise program is one that becomes a lifelong habit. A high school or college athlete who stops exercising in midlife is at greater risk than a person who has always been "only" a walker. It's the old "use it or lose it" adage. Not only will you lose it, it will be bigger, broken down, and less useful when you finally abandon it.

Chapter 6

ARE YOU TOO SHORT
FOR YOUR WEIGHT?

A merica is fighting an obesity epidemic. If being fat were an infectious disease, you would be lining up for your vaccine.

As a country, we were not always obese, but look at the people around you. Americans are big, really big. In fact, more Americans are bigger today than even one generation ago. We've grown accustomed to thinking the people we see today are normal size. They are not. The average American is bigger, and the obese among us are more obese than ever before.

Over the last 50 years, America has witnessed a staggering increase in obesity. In 1950, only 10% of Americans were obese. By 2000, 33% of American adults were obese. In the last 10 years alone, obesity has increased 60%. Today nearly 60 million Americans are obese.[32] Two troubling statistics highlight this crisis:

1. The most obese people are the fastest-growing group. (Pun intended.) In 1990, only 0.8% of the population had a body mass index over 40 (for BMI details, see below). By 2000, this number had nearly tripled to 2.2% of the population.[33]

2. The number of obese children has increased 400% in just
25 years, from 4% of the population in 1980 to an astonishing 15% in 2000. Obese children are condemned to serious health trouble by age 30 or 40. The tragedy is that obese
children will develop health problems only because they are
obese. This is a disaster for the country's future, and it's
unfolding right before our eyes.

WHY WEIGHT MATTERS

Currently, smoking is the number one cause of premature
death at 435,000 deaths each year, but the obese/inactive group is
growing quickly and has already reached 400,000 deaths annually.
In a few years, obesity will replace smoking as the number one
cause of premature death and disease in America.[34]

This chapter will discuss the reasons behind current obesity
epidemic, your body size, how to eat less food, the health risks,
and costs of being overweight or obese. Please keep in mind
that no one is trying to socially stigmatize the obese. Rather,
the focus is to look frankly at the private and public costs of
this epidemic.

Being obese prevents you from achieving good health by
both making you weaker and changing your internal biochemistry. Obesity not only undermines your health, it's also costly
for you, your health insurer, and the financial welfare of the
whole nation.

To understand the role of your weight in your overall health:

1. You need to understand why people have gained weight, so you can avoid the pitfalls as you follow the path to good health.

2. You need to determine your body size and compare it to historical norms. Our great-grandparents would be shocked by the size of today's Americans walking the streets, shopping in stores, and eating in restaurants.

3. You need to understand how obesity jeopardizes your well-being, makes you sick, keeps you ill longer, and causes more disability.

How Did This Happen?

Those of you who are too short for your weight certainly did not start out 20 years ago with the goal of gaining weight. You did it one extra bite at a time. Adding just a few extra calories every snack and every meal of every day, and pretty soon you were too short for your weight.

You became overweight or obese slowly. And our food culture helped you do it. The restaurants served you more food, the portions got larger, the snacks became more frequent, and the foods changed. A hamburger became a bacon cheeseburger. A regular thin-crust pizza turned into a double-cheese stuffed deep-dish pizza. A standard-size soda grew from 12 ounces to 20. The value—lots more food for a little more money—appealed to your sense of thrift: for a few cents more, you could "super-size" your order. Who could resist?

Moreover, you didn't start out to eat primarily processed foods, but as you became busier, they became easier to find and were certainly easier to prepare. Freezer-to-microwave is often the path of least resistance, even if you don't know what the mystery ingredients are.

Over the years, almost like magic, more food just appeared everywhere. On your plate, in your store, in your car, in your cupboard. Food is now available everywhere and anytime—and all served in larger portions.

Thirty years ago, we still ate a healthy diet in reasonable portions. Sometime after that, marketers started pushing sweet carbonated beverages and 32 flavors of chips. Rubber fruit on paper strips (basically corn syrup) became the convenience foods for lunchboxes instead of a bunch of grapes. And fried chips of all flavors, from sour-cream ranch to jalapeno-cheddar, tantalized young and old tastebuds alike. Low-fat diets were promoted as healthy, so no-fat, high-carbohydrate diets became the fad. Then suddenly it was low-carb, high-fat diets. And all of this happened at exactly the same time that we were becoming less physically active. It is little wonder that we lost the battle of the waistline.

Portion sizes have also had a huge impact on our waistlines. To really understand how your food portion sizes have changed in the past few decades, just consider these facts:

Food Yesterday, Food Today

◆ In 1955, the first McDonald's franchise opened. The first drive-through window opened in 1975. Today there are over

10,000 McDonald's restaurants in America and another 20,000 worldwide. Plus thousands more Burger Kings, Pizza Huts, Kentucky Fried Chickens, Taco Bells, Wendy's, Krispy Kremes, and Starbucks.

◆ In 1955, a McDonald's meal was a 3-ounce hamburger, an 8-ounce soda, and a little paper bag with 15 French fries. That was lunch. And, by the way, that is still an acceptable and relatively healthy (fries excepted) lunch—especially compared to everything else around us. Today's Burger King Whopper totals 760 calories, a 300% increase in the hamburger calories alone.

◆ A soda bottle in 1974 held 6.5 ounces and added up to 80 calories. Today's average soda bottle holds 20 ounces of soda and 250 calories. And a Double Gulp at 7-Eleven holds 64 ounces of soda and has 800 calories.

◆ In 1980, a bagel measured 3 inches in diameter and contained 140 calories. Today, it measures 7 inches and has 350 calories, a 250% increase. That's without the added cream cheese.

◆ A muffin of 1980 weighed 2 ounces. Today's muffin is often over 8 ounces.

◆ In 1950, a dinner plate was 10 inches in diameter. Today it is 12 inches in diameter. A 12-inch plate holds substantially more food than a 10-inch plate.

"SUPER-SIZE IT" MARKETING WORKS

Part of your weight problem is that marketing and advertisements really do work. When the processed food people figured out that the food cost was the smallest part of the retail cost, they realized they could sell bigger portions for only a modest increase in price. Everyone loves a bargain, and sales took off. At 7-Eleven, a 16-ounce soda is 5¢ per ounce while a 32-ounce soda is 2.7¢ per ounce. You pay $3.00 for six bagels, but for 50¢ more, you can get a full dozen. Everyone—from fast-food places to candy bar makers to movie theaters—has discovered that if they offer a little bit more food at a slightly higher price, consumers will buy larger portions. And if you have more food in front of you, you will eat more food. More food is more calories. And more calories is added weight.

LABEL MISINFORMATION

Manufacturers are required to put labels on our foods to let us know what we are eating. However, they are not required to follow logic in their labeling practices. The soda bottle says 100 calories per serving, but the bottle contains 2 1/2 servings for a total of 250 calories. The one-pound bag of potato chips? There may be more chips in the bag, but a serving size is still 12 to 15, chips and they still total 120 calories per serving. One of my favorite mislabels was identified by Tara Parker Pope, who writes the "Health Journal" column in the *Wall Street Journal.* She noted that PAM, the cooking spray, identifies itself as "fat free," but in reality is 100% fat. How can this be? It happens because the government defines "fat free" as less than 0.5 gram of fat per serving. The average PAM serving spritz is less than 0.5 grams. Use any more than a little burst of spray, and suddenly it is fat.

Then we have the low-fat or no-fat cookie debacle. "Low fat" sounds healthy, and "no fat" sounds almost virtuous. You may feel more virtuous eating these no-fat cookies, but beware: both the regular and the no-fat versions have nearly the same number of calories. And calories are calories. And added calories is added weight.

SEE MORE, EAT MORE

Food is everywhere, and it's neatly packaged so we can eat while walking or working or talking or sitting in school. The ubiquitous presence of food causes us to eat more. Another reason we eat more? Packages are bigger. Even "small" candy bars are bigger than they used to be. There is a very subtle psychology to larger packages.

This is from the "you gotta love it" research department. Dr. Brian Wansink, a professor of marketing at the University of Illinois, studies why we eat and how much we eat. He went to the theater and gave people either a medium or a large bucket of popcorn. The people with the large bucket consistently ate 50% more than the people with the medium size container. Dr. Wansink repeated the experiment with 14-day-old, stale, theater popcorn—and again, the people with the large bucket ate 30% more than those with the medium container.

He repeated the study with bags of M&M's. He gave people either a 1/2-, 1-, or 2- pound bag of M&M's and a movie video. Then he sent them home to watch the video. When the movie was over, he collected the bags and counted how many M&M's were left. People with the small bag ate 63 M&M's, those with the

1-pound bag ate 120 M&M's, and those with the 2-pound bag ate even more.

He has conducted this same experiment with everything from soup to all-you-can-eat buffets. Yet there is a silver lining in all this: if you give someone a large bowl of carrots, he or she will also eat more carrots.[35]

Grabbing that extra handful of chips or cookies adds up. Eating even slightly larger portions of food adds up. But often we do not just eat "a little" more. The portions around us are often absolutely, unforgivingly huge. So we eat more. And when we eat more of a very high-calorie food, we really eat a lot of calories.

Where are the calories hiding?

◆ One cup of ice cream contains 200 calories. A one-cup dish of premium ice cream contains 300 calories. An ice cream from Cold Stone Creamery with toppings can often total more than 1,000 calories.

◆ Think your frozen yogurt from TCBY has fewer calories? Frozen yogurt is lower in fat than ice cream but has almost the same number of calories. TCBY also knows how to add calories to yogurt. A TCBY Toffee Coffee Cappuccino Chiller has 1,200 calories.[36]

◆ Black coffee has no calories, but a Starbucks 16-ounce latte made with low-fat milk has 220 calories. Heaven forbid you have their great-looking carrot cake with your coffee. That carrot cake alone is another 600 calories.

◆ A Burger King Whopper with cheese has 800 calories. The large fries are another 450.

◆ Even a steady stream of little things count—10 easy-to-eat Hershey kisses total 230 calories.

◆ An 8-ounce serving of potato chips totals 1,200 calories.

◆ A jumbo tub of movie popcorn without extra butter has 1,600 calories. And that's without the additional calories of the butter-flavored mystery fat or a jumbo sugared soda.

All of these changes have enticed us to eat, on average, 300 more calories a day than we did just a decade ago. These extra calories add up quickly. It takes only 3,500 extra calories to add one pound. At 300 added calories a day, you'll gain one extra pound every 12 days. Or 30 pounds per year. It is a wonder we all do not weigh even more.

So while our dietary national disaster is not entirely our fault, it is now our problem and, maybe, your problem.

ARE YOU TOO SHORT FOR YOUR WEIGHT?

Science now measures body weight, not as pounds and inches, but rather as a single number called the body mass index, the BMI, which applies to both men and women. This is a single calculated number that correlates your weight and your height. This single number measures body fat and takes into consideration different heights. Your health, for better or worse, correlates closely with your BMI.

Here's how to determine your body mass index, BMI. First weigh yourself and measure your height without shoes. Then either look at the table below or search for BMI calculators on the Internet.

For the mathematically inclined, BMI is calculated as weight in kilograms divided by height in meters squared. For the metric-phobic, the BMI can be calculated as your weight in pounds times 703 divided by your height in inches squared. For the rest of us, just look at the table below. If you are not on the table below, search the Internet by typing "calculate BMI" into your search engine.

Dennis stands 6'0" tall and weighs 175 pounds. His BMI is 23.7, and according to the federal classification, he has a normal BMI, with the lowest risk of disease.

His friend Philip is 6'0" but weighs 280 pounds. His BMI is 38.0, and he falls into the obese class II category, with a very high risk of disease.

Susan stands 5'4" and weights 136 pounds. Her BMI is 23.3, almost exactly the same as her husband, Dennis, who is 8 inches taller. Despite their height differences, they have the same amount of body fat, relatively speaking. Susan has the same medical risks as her husband, Dennis.

Philip's wife, Diane, is also 5'4", but she weighs 192 pounds. Her BMI is 33. She is in the obese category and has extra health risks.

Once you've found your BMI, compare it to the body mass index definitions below. Note the federal government developed these category labels after identifying the group with the lowest mortality.

Table 14 CLASSIFICATION OF BMI		
Definition and criteria of BMI used by the National Institutes of Health	BMI	Health risk
Underweight	Less than 18.5	Slightly increased
Normal weight	18.5 to 24.9	Lowest
Overweight	25 to 29.9	Increasing
Moderate obesity, Class I	30 to 34.9	High
Severe obesity, Class II	35 to 39.9	Very high
Morbid obesity, Class III	Above 40	Extremely high

WHAT THE NUMBERS MEAN

Your BMI must be interpreted in the context of your overall health.

◆ A person with a BMI under 18.5, the underweight category, can be quite healthy or quite ill, depending on why the weight is so low. You have no increased risk if your BMI has been stable for several years. On the other hand, your risk is substantial if you have emphysema from smoking or a recent unexplained weight loss.

Table 13

BODY MASS INDEX

Note: This table applies to adults ages 18 and over. There are separate BMI tables for children at

BMI	19	20	21	22	23	24	25	26	27	28	29
Height (ft.,in.)					Body Weight (pounds)						
4' 10"	91	96	100	105	110	115	119	124	129	134	138
4' 11"	94	99	104	109	114	119	124	128	133	138	143
5'	97	102	107	112	118	123	128	133	138	143	148
5' 1"	100	106	111	116	122	127	132	137	143	148	153
5' 2"	104	109	115	120	126	131	136	142	147	153	158
5' 3"	107	113	118	124	130	135	141	146	152	158	163
5' 4"	110	116	122	128	134	140	145	151	157	163	169
5' 5"	114	120	126	132	138	144	150	156	162	168	174
5' 6"	118	124	130	136	142	148	155	161	167	173	179
5' 7"	121	127	134	140	146	153	159	166	172	178	185
5' 8"	125	131	138	144	151	158	164	171	177	184	190
5' 9"	128	135	142	149	155	162	169	176	182	189	196
5' 10"	132	139	146	153	160	167	174	181	188	195	202
5' 11"	136	143	150	157	165	172	179	186	193	200	208
6'	140	147	154	162	169	177	184	191	199	206	213
6' 1"	144	151	159	166	174	182	189	197	204	212	219
6' 2"	148	155	163	171	179	186	194	202	210	218	225
6' 3"	152	160	168	176	184	192	200	208	216	224	232
6' 4"	156	164	172	180	189	197	205	213	221	230	238

http://www.cdc.gov/nccdphp/dnpa/bmi/bmi-for-age.htm. It is quicker to type "BMI for children" into your search engine.

30	31	32	33	34	35	36	37	38	39	40	41	42
143	148	153	158	162	167	172	177	181	186	191	196	201
148	153	158	163	168	173	178	183	188	193	198	203	208
153	158	163	168	174	179	184	189	194	199	204	209	215
158	164	169	174	180	185	190	195	201	206	211	217	222
164	169	175	180	186	191	196	202	207	213	218	224	229
169	175	180	186	191	197	203	208	214	220	225	231	237
174	180	186	192	197	204	209	215	221	227	232	238	244
180	186	192	198	204	210	216	222	228	234	240	246	252
186	192	198	204	210	216	223	229	235	241	247	253	260
191	198	204	211	217	223	230	236	242	249	255	261	268
197	203	210	216	223	230	236	243	249	256	262	269	276
203	209	216	223	230	236	243	250	257	263	270	277	284
209	216	222	229	236	243	250	257	264	271	278	285	292
215	222	229	236	243	250	257	265	272	279	286	293	301
221	228	235	242	250	258	265	272	279	287	294	302	309
227	235	242	250	257	265	272	280	288	295	302	310	318
233	241	249	256	264	272	280	287	295	303	311	319	326
240	248	256	264	272	279	287	295	303	311	319	327	335
246	254	263	271	279	287	295	304	312	320	328	336	344

◆ A BMI between 18.5 and 25 is considered normal because this group has the lowest risk of disease. However, even a normal BMI will not save an inactive smoker who eats all the wrong foods.

◆ A person with a BMI in the 26 to 27 range who is otherwise very fit and eats well has only a minimal increase in risk. But if your BMI is 27 and you have been a couch potato, you can expect to gain weight soon. Then your troubles will really accumulate along with the added pounds.

◆ As your BMI moves above 28, health problems start to occur solely because you are too heavy.

◆ As your BMI rises above 30, your risk of a serious future disease increases significantly. By the time your BMI is 35, the risk to your health is the same as if you smoked a pack of cigarettes a day. If your BMI is over 40, your risk of a serious future disease is all but certain.

◆ BMI is even an accurate predictor for professional athletes. The BMI and mortality of 6,800 football players has been studied. Professional players have a BMI ranging from roughly 24 for field goal kickers to 27 for quarterbacks to 38 or more for linemen. Football players who are not obese have better mortality than the general population. However, linemen with a BMI over 32 had a rate of cardiovascular death six times higher than the players with a BMI under 28.[37]

Janet was a motivated mother of three children. She and her husband both worked two jobs to give their children the opportunity for a college education. For almost 10 years, Janet ate fast food two or three times a day because of her busy schedule. And her body showed it. Janet weighed nearly 230 pounds, yet she stood only 5'3". She was indeed too short—way too short—for her weight.

At an Educational Hour lecture on obesity at her church, Janet learned she had a body mass index of 40.7. After the talk, she and her friends chatted over pastries during the church coffee hour.

But Janet was bothered. She had not felt well the past few months. She was sluggish and short of breath, and even simple chores left her fatigued.

YOUR WAIST SIZE ALSO MATTERS

If you are overweight or obese, the other important measurement to watch is the size of your waist. If you carry your extra weight in your belly, you are at greater risk for future health problems than if you carry your extra weight around your hips. These two weight patterns are often referred to as apple and pear body shapes.

To find out which shape you are, measure your waist. Wrap a string or a paper tape measure around your waist. Measure your waist *at the level of your navel.* Sorry, guys, you cannot use your belt size as your waist size. Many of you wear your belt far below your waist.

Obese men with a waist more than 40 inches and obese women with a waist over 35 inches have a greatly increased risk of type 2 diabetes and aggressive heart disease. These waist measurements indicate an even higher risk than predicted by a high BMI alone. Large waist measurements are associated with the Metabolic Syndrome (see below).

Dennis stands 6'0" tall and weighs 175 pounds. His BMI is 23.7. His waist measures 35 inches. He is at a normal weight and at the lowest risk for disease.

His friend, Philip, is 6'0" but weighs 280 pounds. His BMI is 38.0. His waist measures 46 inches. Given his BMI alone, Philip is at high risk, but his waist measurement of over 40 inches puts him at an even higher level of risk.

Susan stands 5'4" and weighs 136 pounds. Her BMI is 23.3, and her waist is 29 inches. She is at very low risk.

Philip's wife, Diane, is also 5'4" but she weighs 192 pounds. Her BMI is 33. Her waist measures 38 inches. She is at very high risk based on both her BMI and her waist measurement.

THE METABOLIC SYNDROME ADDS EXTRA RISK

The Metabolic Syndrome is a high-risk condition that signals the impending dangers of aggressive heart disease and type 2 diabetes. Abdominal fat does not just sit there passively. Abdominal fat is metabolically active fat. What does that mean?

From the close-enough-translation-of-science department comes this analogy to explain insulin resistance. Abdominal fat is an active fat. It both absorbs insulin the way a sponge absorbs water and secretes hormones that increase cardiovascular inflammation.

When a thin person eats, his or her blood sugar rises and the pancreas produces insulin, which forces the blood sugar into cells; the blood sugar level falls back to normal, and the pancreas rests. But when an obese person eats, his or her blood sugar rises, and the pancreas produces insulin, which is absorbed by the abdominal fat. So the blood sugar stays high and the pancreas goes into high gear and stays there, trying to produce enough insulin.

The obese person's situation is like driving your car as fast as it will go without changing the oil. Eventually both your car engine and your pancreas burn out. As the insulin-producing cells of your pancreas start to burn out, you become pre-diabetic, and once they are burned out, you are diabetic. Even the best pills for diabetes do not return you to normal health. The only remedy is prevention: lose weight before you develop insulin resistance, glucose intolerance, or diabetes.

In addition, abdominal fat produces harmful changes to your blood cholesterols. In general, the good HDL cholesterol falls, the bad LDL cholesterol rises, and triglycerides increase. Abdominal fat also produces both inflammatory and oxidative chemicals to further stress your body chemistry and the fragile lining of your arteries.

Table 15 THE METABOLIC SYNDROME IS DIAGNOSED WHEN YOU MEET THREE OF THE FIVE CRITERIA	
Waist measurement	Men: more than 40 inches Women: more than 35 inches
Triglycerides	More than 150
HDL cholesterol (the good kind)	Men: less than 40 Women: less than 50
Blood pressure	Greater than 130/80
Fasting blood sugar	Greater than 110

OBESITY IS A DISEASE

Obesity is a very dangerous disease. Being obese increases your health risks. A person with a BMI over 35 shares the same health risk as someone who smokes a pack of cigarettes per day. Excess weight accounts for an additional 300,000 to 400,000 unnecessary and premature deaths per year.

The current national obesity epidemic will burden the nation with a tremendous health crisis in future years. Obesity is closely linked to major chronic degenerative diseases that gobble up medical resources. Here are some scientific facts to put the health risks of obesity in perspective.

Being obese shortens your life expectancy. The famous Framingham Heart Study found that 40-year-old people with a BMI of 26–29 died 3 years sooner than those with a BMI less than 25. Those with a BMI of 30 or more died 7 years sooner.[38]

The American Cancer Society studied the risk of death of

1,000,000 Americans by body mass index.[39] Their results are shown in the graph below. The people with the lowest mortality had a BMI between 20 and 24.9. Note how quickly the risk of death rises when the BMI climbs above 28.0. The chart shows that people with a BMI of 40 are three times more likely to die than those with a BMI between 20 and 27.9.

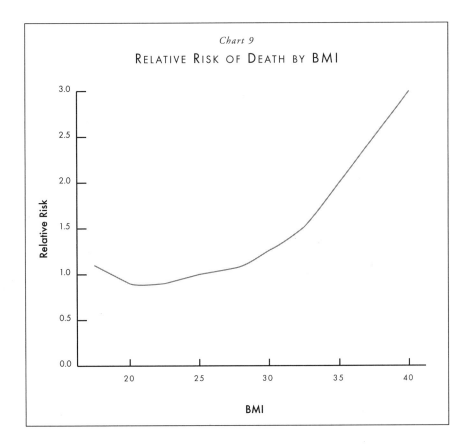

Chart 9
RELATIVE RISK OF DEATH BY BMI

◆ **Obesity causes type 2 diabetes**. And the more obese you are, the higher the risk of diabetes.[40] People with a BMI of 40 or greater have a 750% increase in the risk of developing diabetes compared to a thin person.[41] The association is so strong that some experts now refer to obesity and diabetes as one epidemic, diabesity.

◆ **Obesity is linked with more than 80% of all cases of type 2 diabetes in both children and adults.** Preventing diabetes is more powerful than treating diabetes. More than 80% of all type 2 diabetes can be prevented by weight loss and exercise. Despite medical therapy, diabetes remains a leading cause of blindness, kidney failure, heart disease, amputations, and premature death.

◆ **Obesity is clearly linked with heart disease.** Obesity raises the bad LDL cholesterol, lowers the good HDL cholesterol, increases blood triglycerides, raises markers of inflammation, and elevates blood pressure. The Nurses' Health Study studied 115,000 women over 16 years. Even looking at women who had never smoked, the risk of cardiovascular disease was more than four times greater in women with a BMI over 32 than in women with a BMI under 25.[42]

◆ **Obesity is linked with about 20% of all cancers.** The National Cancer Institute estimates that obesity and inactivity may account for 25% to 30% of all cancers, including cancer of the colon and breast. The NCI also estimates that 14% of all cancer deaths in men and 20% in women were due to obesity.[43] At the 11th European Congress on Obesity, experts noted that we could reduce the number of cancers by 30% or 40% by better diets, more exercise, and less obesity.

◆ **Obesity in children is particularly troubling.** Many obese children already have the biological markers for cardiovascular disease, hypertension, and diabetes. Up to 4% of obese adolescents now have type 2 diabetes, and in some clinics, they represent half of all new cases.[44] Many more will develop obesity-caused type 2 diabetes in their 20s or 30s. Until this recent obesity epidemic, type 2 diabetes in children was unheard of in the world of pediatrics. These children will be condemned to live with the complications of what is basically a preventable disease.

OBESITY COSTS SERIOUS MONEY

Obesity costs money, jaw-dropping amounts of money. The costs are directly proportional to the amount of excess weight an individual has amassed. Neither a private insurance company nor Medicaid will be able to control health care costs if obesity continues to be rampant.

The Centers for Disease Control[45] reports:

◆ In 2000, the total cost of obesity in the United States was $117 billion—$61 billion in direct medical costs and $56 billion in indirect costs.

◆ In 1997–1999, annual hospital costs related to childhood and adolescent obesity totaled $127 million, up from $35 million in 1979–1981.

◆ Among U.S. adults in 1996, cardiovascular disease related to overweight and obesity cost $31 billion.

◆ In the Swedish Obesity Study, obese people took twice the number of sick days as people of normal weight. Obese people were also 2 1/2 times more likely to draw a disability pension.[46]

Back to Janet.

> The guest speaker at the church education hour had also mentioned waist measurements during the lecture on obesity. At home, Janet took her tailor's tape measure, gritted her teeth, and measured her waist. Janet's waist was 38 inches. According to the information on the handout Janet got at the meeting, Janet should see her physician to be checked for all of the complications of obesity and diabetes. Janet was beginning to regret going to the church Educational Hour.
>
> Janet's physician scared her with "all his talk about diabetes and high blood pressure and heart disease." Having recently buried her father, Janet listened. For the first time, she understood. Everything taken together meant she was unequivocally obese and showing early signs of medical complications stemming from her obesity.
>
> Janet knew she had to change or plan on joining her father sooner than she wanted. The only question: how to change. All of her prior diets had been short-lived, and they had failed miserably.

DOES LOSING WEIGHT MATTER?

By now, you know that obesity is unhealthy. The question that remains is whether or not weight loss can make a difference. Once again, there is good scientific data in the affirmative.

One study of almost 30,000 overweight women found that intentional weight loss of more than 20 pounds (9.1 kg) was associated with a 25% decrease in death rates, including both cardiovascular and cancer deaths.[47]

The same study looked carefully at the 15,000 women who already had medical complications such as diabetes or heart disease. In this group, *any* weight loss was associated with a 10% reduction in cardiovascular disease and a 20% reduction in death from any cause, primarily due to a reduction in mortality from obesity-related cancer.[48]

WHAT CAN YOU DO TO LOSE WEIGHT?

Calories are calories. Your weight is not determined by the kinds of food you eat. Your weight is the total number of calories you eat compared to the number of calories you burn in exercise. And right now, the national scale is tipped with exercise down on one side, and calories and weight way up on the other.

Dr. Bob says:

♦ *Successful weight loss requires both eating less and exercising more. One will not work without the other.*

To rebalance the scale requires a clear three-part approach: exercise more, eat less, and eat healthier foods. Chapter 5 covered the importance of exercise. This chapter will discuss how to eat fewer calories. Chapter 7 will focus on how to eat healthier foods.

Diets work in the short term because any diet that permits only some foods and limits others helps you limit total calories. The very popular low-carb diets of today work because they really force you to avoid snacks, most of which are empty carbohydrates and fats. These diets suggest menus limiting calories to under 2,000 per day.

All diets, unfortunately, fail in the long term. We can eat only so much grapefruit or boiled eggs or steaks topped with whipped cream without going craving crazy. Five years after starting a diet, 90% of dieters are back at their starting weight, if not more than their starting weight.

The only way to succeed in losing weight and keeping it off for the long term is to reduce the number of calories you take in. This also means you almost always have to change what you eat. You cannot simply eat less of everything you ate yesterday. Part of the reason you ate too much was that the food you were eating was nutritionally empty and not satisfying. So your goal is to eat smarter.

If you spend time in a cafeteria or at a buffet, you can learn a great deal by watching people's plates. The plates of people who are lean look very different from the plates of people who are obese. A lean person will make a salad of spinach, tomatoes, carrots, cucumber, raisins, sesame seeds, and a healthy splash of olive oil and vinegar. An obese person will make a chef's salad with iceberg lettuce, cheese, and ham—and then drench the whole thing in fat-free dressing. The obese person built a salad using nutritionally empty lettuce, too many high-fat ingredients, and to top it off, fat-free salad dressing, which usually has as many calories as regular salad dressing.

The same lesson is repeated over and over, regardless of where you turn. Watch a lean and an obese person eat at a fast-food restaurant. The lean person will order a hamburger, a bowl of soup, and a diet soda. You guessed it: the obese person will order a super-size double-bacon cheeseburger, with fries and soda. Time and time again. Go to the movies. Small popcorn, no butter versus jumbo popcorn, extra butter.

Right away Janet decided she needed to eat better. This turned out to be harder than she thought. It was impossible to eat just half of a double cheeseburger and large fries.

First, she had to move from cheeseburgers to a hamburger, from double-crust pizza to thin-crust-light-on-the-cheese pizza. Actually, just going from two cheeseburgers to two hamburgers was relatively easy. And that single change saved her 100 calories every day.

Quietly over the next year, she changed her diet. She began to order a hamburger instead of a cheeseburger and a diet soda instead of a regular soda. Her cupboards at home were still stocked with chips and cookies. The weight loss process was difficult; she joined Weight Watchers for the support and advice the organization provided.

It took more than six months, but Weight Watchers helped her move further: to a portion-size grilled chicken salad with a diet soda. She brought fruit from home as a snack instead of store-bought cookies. The foods in her cupboards began to change. In fact, her cupboard looked almost empty, but she was not hungry, and her husband had not complained—well, not too loudly.

Just as eating half of a double cheeseburger didn't work, Janet found that eating fewer cookies didn't work either. She used to love a handful of cookies. She tried munching just two at a time, but she found her willpower too weak. The only solution? Not keeping the cookies in the house. That seemed to work.

Janet also wanted to exercise. The gym was out both for lack of time and confidence. So she added little bits of walking while trying to find an exercise she liked. At first, all that she did was park farther away from work. She tried to walk a little faster each time she walked. Soon she was walking a fast-paced 45 minutes a day.

So if eating less and eating better is the trick to long-term weight loss, how do you do it? First, you have to know what you eat. Next, you have to understand how much food you are eating. It is very possible to eat very good food and lose weight. You may eat even better food in your new diet than in your old. Eating well to lose weight certainly does not have to be a sacrifice.

How to Start: Practice Safe Eating

The only way to lose weight is to both eat fewer calories and get more exercise. And with that, you roll your eyes. You were hoping for a miracle diet. Will you settle for knowing what it takes to eat sensibly? If you can start to learn this, the results could be miraculous. These rules will start you eating less and eating better.

At the get-go, you should know I am not a diet expert, so I'm not going to focus on either the highly popular low-carb or low-fat diets. But the truth is that I have watched too many people go to a low-fat diet. They feel virtuous as they eat large portions of low- or no-fat foods, often containing the same total number of calories as the high-fat version. And that is not a diet. At the same time, I watch friends go on the low-carb diet and switch to sausage and cheese for breakfast. Guaranteed, this is not a healthy diet. They may lose weight. They may watch their cholesterol drop initially—but cholesterols always drop as you lose weight. And when they start to cheat by adding carbs, their cholesterols go crazy. This is not a diet for long-term health.

My real lesson for you is this: to lose or control your weight, first, eat less food. Second, eliminate the highly processed junk foods from your diet. Third, eat better food. Chapter 7 will focus on scientifically proven health-promoting foods. But before you discover those foods, you have to learn how much food you eat and start to eat less. Even 10% less food is a great start.

HOW TO EAT LESS

The next seven "practice safe eating" rules are quite powerful and will help you reduce the number of calories you eat. I want you to follow these rules to help you eat less and better.

1. Keep a food diary for a week.

I strongly suggest you keep a food diary for one week. Write down what and when you eat. If you are honest with yourself, you will be astonished at what and when you really eat during the week. At the end of the week, you can shred the diary, so no one will see it, but do try to be honest with yourself. Studies indicate that you will underestimate what you eat, and the more obese you are, the more you will underestimate. Even this recognition becomes part of the solution.

Record the details. This means that your lunchtime entry cannot read "ham sandwich." How big was the sandwich? White bread or whole wheat? One or two tablespoons of mayonnaise? One slice of ham, or was it four slices? With two slices of cheese? As you learn to recognize portions, write down the portion sizes of what you eat. Write down the times when you ate or activities that accompanied your eating. Many overweight people eat and snack at night while watching television—another reason to turn off the television and go for a walk. After a week, the foods and the patterns will jump off the page at you. And then you can start to change.

2. Be aware of what you are eating.

Many people, including me, eat nutritionally empty junk foods some of the time. Other people eat a lot of these junk foods a lot of the time. Others eat nutritionally empty foods most of the time.

We are surrounded with convenience foods, processed foods, fast foods, cellophane-wrapped foods. Most of them are devoid of anything good for our health. Some of these convenience foods are flagrantly unhealthy. There is always a healthier option. The only way to really tell the difference is to read the labels.

Next time you are going to eat something ask: Is this food good or bad for my health? The answer does not always have to be super healthy. Everyone has a favorite junk food. But when you eat, be aware of what you are eating. Your diet will change as you start to think about the foods you eat.

3. Be aware of how much you are eating.

Americans no longer know how big a normal-size meal should be. Worse, they often think a portion is whatever is on their plate. As a nation, we seem to have decided that more food means better food. So lots more food must mean really good food. Portions have doubled or tripled in the past 20 years. It is not just in the fast-food restaurants. We have also tripled the amount of food we serve in our own homes.

This excess food is killing us, literally. Bigger does not mean better. Eating more sensible portions of more healthy food is a key to long-term weight control. So, to start, you have to learn what a normal portion size is. It is a whole lot smaller than you think. If we want to get to and maintain a normal weight, we have to eat the same portions we ate in 1980 or even 1970.

Quick serving size comparisons:

◆ A serving of meat is three ounces, about the size of a deck of cards. That 24-ounce steak on your platter? It's really eight portions.

◆ A serving of carbohydrates, such as potatoes or pasta, should be close to the size of a tennis ball. Not the tennis ball can, just a tennis ball.

◆ Many fresh fruits and vegetables often come "prepackaged" by Nature in correct serving sizes. The serving size of an orange is an orange. The serving size of a tomato is one tomato. On the other hand, a serving size of watermelon is not the whole melon; a serving of melon is still the size of an orange.

◆ A serving of ice cream is the size of a tennis ball.

Then to further complicate things, prepackaged food is often disguised as a single serving but contains more than one serving. For example, many people will drink a 20-ounce soda. Remember: that soda is 2 1/2 servings.

Practical applications:

◆ For one week, study portion sizes. Think about what you are eating as a portion size. Is the food on your plate close to a portion size? If not, why not?

◆ Learn how many portions are in a package. Then gradually start to make a choice closer to a correct portion size. You will not achieve portion control overnight.

◆ Pour your usual size bowl of cereal. Now measure it. Then compare your cereal bowl with the recommended portion size on the side of the box. Take your normal evening handful or two of cookies from the bag, count them, now look at the side of the bag to find out how many cookies equal one serving. Read how many calories are in that portion.

◆ Eat close to a correct portion size. This means:

• A normal-size bagel is 3 inches in diameter. If your bagel outlet serves only 7-inch bagels, buy one, give half to a friend, or save the other half for tomorrow. At half a 7-inch bagel, you are still eating more than a portion size.

• A portion-size and acceptable fast-food meal is a regular hamburger at McDonald's along with a diet soda and a salad.

- When you buy a chicken breast for dinner, remember that is dinner for two. And the pasta serving should be only about a cupful.

- Your new portion sizes look awfully puny on your typical 12-inch dinner plate. Consider buying 10-inch dinner plates.

- When you go to the movies, buy a small popcorn. No extra butter. No refills.

◆ Do not cook large amounts of food. Learn to cook smaller portions of better quality foods. If you cook too much, immediately put the leftovers into the freezer.

◆ Do not buy huge portions of food. You will just feel compelled to eat more. That goes for buying the jumbo bag of cookies, too. You will eat more cookies just because there are more cookies.

◆ Do not eat food from the bag. You will have no idea how many portions you have eaten.

4. Order and eat responsibly in restaurants.

We love to eat out. And restaurants love to feed us. They serve huge portions. A restaurant meal contains at least a couple hundred calories more than the same meal prepared at home. If a restaurant puts huge portions on your plate and you eat them, where do you think the calories go? Until restaurants learn to serve reasonable amounts of food, you have to protect yourself.

Practical applications:

◆ Order sensibly. This means:

- Forget about the 24-ounce steak. If the restaurant offers four sizes of steak, work your way down gradually.

- Tell the server, no fries. Remember, you have no willpower. You do not even want fries on your plate. If the server brings you fries by mistake, send them back.

- Order appetizers as your entrée. Order a salad or soup as your first course.

- Split the dish with your significant other. Just tip the server extra for the meal you did not order.

◆ Never eat super-size anything.

◆ Do not even go the restaurant that offers jumbo everything or the all-you-can-eat buffet. No one has that much willpower.

Dr. Bob says:

◆ *Your mother was wrong. You do not have to clean your plate.*

5. Eat deep-fried foods rarely.

Deep-fried foods are cooked in the very worst kinds of fat and are loaded with calories. These foods taste good and are a real part of our culture. You can eat them but do so rarely.

Practical application:

◆ Make French fries, deep-fried clams, fried chicken, and doughnuts a rare treat, not an ordinary food.

◆ Do not eat chips. Eat nuts instead. This choice trades an unhealthy fat for a healthy fat.

6. Push back.

Don't be afraid to push back from the table after you have eaten a portion-size meal. This will give your brain time to get the message that you just ate. Some people have lost the sense of what it means to have eaten enough. This is a difficult sensation to find again if you have lost it. So learn to push way back away from the table rather than go back for seconds.

Practical application:

- ◆ Fill 2/3 of your 10-inch plate with colorful vegetables. Then add your meat and a carbohydrate course. That is dinner. When you are finished, push back. Leave the table if you must. Don't go back for second servings for at least 20 minutes. This will give your brain time to get the message that you have eaten.

- ◆ Eat something like a handful of nuts about half an hour before you eat a meal or go grocery shopping. This will calm your hunger and may start to send signals to your brain that you are full or not so hungry.

- ◆ Eat more slowly and mindfully. Enjoy the food you eat. Eating should not be a competitive sport.

7. Eat dessert only on rare occasions.

Desserts taste good. And they are loaded with calories. You certainly do not need dessert after every meal.

Practical application:

- ◆ Do not order a high-fat, high-calorie dessert even to share. You know you will eat most of it.

◆ Do not think frozen yogurt has fewer calories than the ice cream. It doesn't.

◆ Eat fresh fruit as dessert whenever possible. Many restaurants have fresh fruit year round. They can easily make you a small bowl.

◆ When at a restaurant and you really want dessert, your second choice is a fruit pie, fruit crisp, or crumble. Just do not eat the crust. All right, just not all of the crust.

Janet's weight slowly began to drop. A steady pound a week or so. After two years, Janet weighed 165 pounds, and her body mass index was down to 29. She felt fabulous on her new diet and her new way of living.

Even though Janet's body mass index was still at the border between overweight and obese, she looked wonderful and felt really healthy. Her physician was mightily impressed. All of her borderline blood sugar, blood pressure, and cholesterols were now close to normal. Janet found she could lose weight and keep it off. Not only by eating less, *but by eating differently.*

In fact, everyone loved the new Janet except her church group. Janet was now the thinnest person in it. Their social pressure was anything but subtle. Janet valued her friends but knew the importance of her own future health. When she attended meetings, she chose the smallest piece of cake, which she thoroughly enjoyed with black coffee.

Putting America on a portion-controlled diet will take us part of the way toward better health. This is a good and necessary start. As you look for ways to practice safe eating, you will find yourself wondering what to buy for the fridge, what to serve for dinner, and what to eat.

The chapter you just finished focused on the negative side of food, the too much of all the wrong kinds of food. The next chapter will explore a different and new side of food: food to promote health. Food can be more than calories. Food can and should be very tasty and good for you. Eating the right foods will promote your good health and help you achieve your goal of living actively for a long time.

Chapter 7

LIFE IS TOO SHORT
FOR FAST FOOD

To get us started and thinking about your diet, let's take another one of my unscientific quizzes.

		Self-assessment 2 WHAT COLOR IS YOUR DIET?	
	Disease-promoting way of eating	Average diet	Health-promoting way of eating
What kind of food do you eat?	More than half the time I eat fast food or already prepared convenience foods— I'm a busy person. I like to snack, and I eat junk food.	I eat what is near me when I'm hungry without thinking about it.	I consciously choose healthy foods, and I like them.
Fruits and veggies	Does lettuce on my burger or tomato sauce on my pizza count?	1, maybe 2, rarely 3 a day.	At least 5 or 6 a day of varied color.
Whole grains	Not a chance.	An occasional whole-grain breakfast cereal.	2 or more servings per day. I love whole-grain cereals and breads.
Fish	Not unless it's dipped in batter and deep-fried.	Occasionally.	2 or more times a week.
Oils and fats	Crisco, lard, and bacon fat make the best deep-fried chicken.	I don't cook, so I don't know much about oils and fats. I don't know how to tell a bad from a good fat.	I primarily use olive or other liquid vegetable oil.
Snacks	I snack on microwave popcorn with extra butter.	I eat whatever is available in the fridge at home.	I like apples, grapes, or a granola bar. But I stay away from granola bars that contain trans-fatty acids.
Color your diet	White. Filled with white bread, potatoes, lard, microwave popcorn.	Plaid. This diet is a little of this and that. It is also how most people eat.	Colorful with lots of different fruits and vegetables, bright green olive oils, and pink salmon.

People look at food in many different ways. Some spend great amounts of energy fretting about low-carb or low-fat foods. To others, whatever is handy in the freezer or lands on their plate is just fine with them. Others judge food by its convenience: buzz it up and eat it on the run. Some treasure familiarity—they don't try anything new or "strange." For still others, food has to have "lots of taste," which often means salt, fat, or sugar. Some like it hot and spicy. Others like it covered in cheese.

One thing, however, is clear. For all of our strongly held views on food, as a country bursting with an abundance of food and the tastes and traditions of many cultures, what we eat is not working well for us.

Food is and should be more than the sum of carbs and fats. It should be more than just what is on our plate or whatever is convenient. Food is what feeds our bodies, our families, and our souls, for better or for worse. We are creatures of nature, and Mother Nature has figured out how foods close to the earth will sustain us. Food has a job to do, and if we let it, food will keep us healthy.

But in the U.S., food has turned into a business, complete with profit margins and mass production. Much of the processed food we buy in the stores has been designed with bottom lines, shelf life, and convenience in mind. These goals rarely coincide with what our bodies need. We have processed the life out of much of our food, so that it now often promotes disease. And despite our plenty, our bodies are assaulted with bad ingredients while they hunger for the nutrition that Mother Nature provides.

What's "good" nutrition? Good nutrition is eating a wide variety of health-promoting foods in reasonable amounts. Health-promoting foods are tasty, familiar to you, and readily available. You just need to understand what healthy foods are so you can make informed decisions about what you put in your grocery cart. Once you understand the nutritional values of healthy food, your next step is to eat them more often and unhealthy foods less often. Good nutrition and healthy eating are as simple as that. No more diet books, no more fad diets. Just know what foods to eat in reasonable portions.

Which foods promote health? How beneficial are they? Health-promoting foods include colorful fruits and vegetables, whole grains, fish, monosaturated and polyunsaturated oils, nuts and beans, eggs, and modest amounts of alcohol. Every study confirms that people who eat diets based on these foods live better and stay more active longer.

TYPICAL AMERICAN EATING HABITS ARE LETHAL

Many foods in the typical American diet are readily available and slowly lethal. A steady diet of French fries, pastries, chips, and double-cheese pizza with sausage slowly eats away at our health. The majority of heart disease, one-third of all cancers, and virtually all of the current obesity-caused diabetes epidemic stem from what and how much Americans eat.

As a nation, we eat staggering amounts of nutritionally empty food and scant amounts of nutritionally helpful foods. Today, we value food for its convenience, the speed of its preparation, and its quantity rather than its quality and contribution to health.

Charlie hardly ever thought about what he ate. Breakfast at home was only coffee, perhaps a small glass of orange juice, a bowl of the kids' cereal, the kind with chocolate and marshmallows, or white-bread cinnamon toast. If he ate at work, he usually had a Danish from the coffee shop.

Lunch was always a business/social affair. Fortunately, there was a fabulous cafeteria in the neighboring bank building, and he ate there often. Lunch might be the grilled hamburger with American, Swiss, blue, or Cheddar cheese, the new Caesar wrap, or a grilled ham-and-cheese. And always fries and a diet soda. Knowing that vegetables were good for him, Charlie often concocted a salad from the self-serve bar. He would pile on the iceberg lettuce, a few cucumber slices, bacon bits—and then ladle on the Thousand Island dressing. He found it difficult to pass up the dessert.

By about four o'clock Charlie was hungry, so he would have a cookie or candy bar from the vending machine—but only one. (He was, after all, watching what he ate.)

When he got home, he usually had some cheese and crackers or chips with his evening drink. Dinner had become a catch-as-catch-can affair because of the kids' activities. His evening meal might be anything from pizza to take-out fried chicken or something from the freezer. When the family ate at home, his wife always included a vegetable, such as broccoli. About once or twice a month, Charlie would grill chicken or ribs, which were excellent.

After Charlie made certain the kids were finished with their homework, he would treat himself to a bowl, or two, of ice cream, watch the evening news, and turn in for the night.

And so far, so good. He had put on "only" 50 pounds since college and was still in very good physical shape. Charlie read widely, and so he was informed enough to know that some people talked about healthy eating. But he might as well have been reading the Greek alphabet. Charlie had absolutely no clue as to how to go about changing his diet. Frankly, he didn't see the need. He thought his eating habits were quite acceptable.

After all, he ate a couple of vegetables in his salad, stayed with diet soda, and always chose a smaller piece of dessert at lunch. Charlie knew that he could hardly be described as a glutton.

Look at Charlie's eating habits. Can you find anything nutritious in his routine? Anything that will improve his health? This is like looking for Waldo. Oh, there it is, a glass of orange juice and a little broccoli. At the end of the week, Charlie has had only a handful of colorful fruits or vegetables. No fish, no whole grains, no nuts. He has, on the other hand, eaten foods high in saturated fats, lots of processed grains, desserts, and candy bars.

Unfortunately, far too many Americans eat the way Charlie does, and they are just as clueless about what, if anything, is wrong with their eating habits or how to change them.

Life after Atkins, the Zone, and South Beach

Then there are those Americans who spend their whole life changing their eating habits. In an effort to lose weight, they slide from one failed diet to another. Americans spend an estimated $40 billion on diet plans and products annually, all without long-term success.

A few years ago, the craze was the low-fat diet. Manufacturers responded by making a low- or no-fat version of everything from cookies to cream cheese. (Just what is "no-fat cream cheese" made from anyway?) The calories, however, stayed nearly the same; just the fat came out. And then we found out that a low-fat and high-carbohydrate approach may not be good for us at all.

Now the craze is the low-carb, high-fat diet. The stores are filled with low-carb everything, from bread to chips. A 2003 Harris survey reported that 32 million Americans were on some version of the low-carb diet.

These two divergent diet approaches—low-carb or low-fat—preach opposing views about which food is good for your health. Both of these divergent diets help people temporarily lose weight for the same reason: they force dieters to monitor, control, and limit what they eat. Both diets restrict free-range eating. Both diets prohibit the morning doughnut, the afternoon candy bar, the evening chips, and the late-night ice cream.

Both fail in the long term for the same reasons. The diets do not focus on portion sizes, do not teach a method to control the number of calories consumed, and do not instruct the dieter about the value of health-promoting foods.

To be successful, a diet must not be a diet. It must a become a long-term lifestyle choice, and it must be healthy. Most people do not know where to turn when it comes time to move off the low-fat or low-carb diet and adopt a long-term maintenance plan. What do they do? They heave a sigh of relief that the diet's over, and they return to their old ways of eating and snacking and gaining weight. They forget—or never realized—that they lost weight because they tightly controlled what and when they ate.

In Search of Healthy Foods

Science has been looking for an optimal approach to eating for decades, and the search is succeeding. Researchers are beginning to understand the differences between a healthy and unhealthy diet. They are defining both the kinds of food associated with premature disease and the kinds of foods associated with less disease and better health. The findings among studies are remarkably consistent.

Large research studies followed hundreds of thousands people for several years: the Nurses' Health Study, the Iowa Women's Health Study, the Seventh Day Adventist Study, the European EPIC study, Lyon Heart Diet Study, and the Okinawa Centenarian Study. All of the data from these studies point in the same general direction.

Everyone agrees: an unhealthy diet is a leading cause of our high rates of heart disease, cancer, and diabetes. There is near-universal agreement about what an unhealthy, disease-promoting eating regimen looks like: it looks like a typical American way of eating.

This unhealthy diet gets the majority, if not all, of its daily calories from:

◆ highly saturated (animal) fats, like butter and partially hydrogenated fats (those hidden in chips, French fries, and store-bought cookies)

◆ highly refined carbohydrates (often found as refined white flour in breads, bagels, and pretzels)

◆ sodas and soft drinks

◆ processed, prepared foods (think frozen cheese-filled thick crust sausage pizza)

While this approach to eating is high in all of the "bad" foods, it also lacks any of the "good" foods.

These same studies identify the foods that promote good health and reduce the risk of disease. The health-promoting foods that we all should eat more often include:

◆ colorful fruits and vegetables

◆ whole grains

◆ nuts

◆ plant-based oils, such as olive or soybean

◆ fish

A 1950s INTERNATIONAL STUDY FOCUSED ON DIET AND HEALTH

In the early 1950s, Dr. Ancel Keyes, a University of Minnesota epidemiologist, began to think about the huge differences among rates of cardiovascular death and disease in countries around the world. He hypothesized that different diets might cause cardiovascular disease.

In his famous study, the Seven Countries Study, Dr. Keyes found several fascinating bits of information, among them:

◆ The low-risk countries of Italy, Greece, and Japan had only 12% to 20% of the risk of coronary artery disease that the high-risk countries, Finland and the United States, had.

◆ Cholesterol levels alone accounted for more than 40% of the cardiovascular disease difference among countries. The combination of high blood pressure and high cholesterol accounted for 60% of the differences between countries.

◆ The strongest link to heart disease was the type of fat rather than the amount of fat consumed. Finland, with the highest consumption of saturated fats (beef and butter) had more heart disease, and Crete with the highest consumption of olive oil, had less heart disease than Keyes had predicted.

This 1950s study correctly identified the islands near Greece as having one of the diets that actually promoted health. Multiple studies involving hundreds of thousands of people have confirmed that eating regimens similar to Greece's will reduce heart disease, stroke, hypertension, diabetes, and many cancers. This diet has been called the Mediterranean diet. All of these studies consistently identify the same foods as promoting health.

LATER STUDIES SUPPORT THE MEDITERRANEAN DIET

The studies below confirm the value of the health-promoting Mediterranean diet. Look carefully at each study. The benefits of this diet are huge.

◆ The Nurses' Health Study confirms that heart disease rates can be reduced 80% by adopting a Mediterranean diet and making lifestyle changes.[49]

◆ A 2002 Mayo Clinic talk summarized the Mediterranean findings well. In a period of eight years, men with diets high in vegetables, fruit, tomatoes, fish, garlic, chicken, and whole grain and low in red meat, processed meat, refined grains, French fries, sweets and desserts, snacks, margarines, and butter had half the heart disease of men with diets showing the opposite patterns.[50]

◆ A recent study from the Harvard School of Public Health echoed the Crete findings when it compared the health of people who ate the typical Western diet with those who ate a more Mediterranean diet. Data showed that men who consumed a typical Western diet were 60% more likely to develop diabetes than those whose diets centered on vegetables, fruits, whole grains, fish, and poultry.[51]

Table 16 COMPARISON OF THE TYPICAL WESTERN AND MEDITERRANEAN DIET	
Western Diet	Mediterranean Diet
Red meat	Vegetables
Processed meat	Fruit
French fries	Fish
High-fat dairy products	Whole grains
Refined grains	Poultry
Sweets and desserts	

◆ The Lyon Heart Diet Study has reported that people who followed a Mediterranean diet for 5 years experienced a 50% lower rate of cancer cases and deaths. The comparison group with a higher rate of cancer ate a diet similar to the American Heart Association diet.[52]

◆ The National Cancer Institute estimates that up to 30% of many cancers may be due to diet.[53]

These tremendous health gains occurred by following a diet high in colorful fruits and vegetables, beans and nuts, fish, and olive and canola oils. This healthy diet is almost the exact opposite of the typical unhealthy American diet.

In addition, the Mediterranean approach to eating can help you lose weight. Other studies have found that people who follow the Mediterranean diet can and do effectively lose weight and keep it off.[54] This approach is really more an informed way of eating than a "diet." You can stick with this way of eating because it is nutritionally balanced, tastes good, and is very satisfying.

So the question becomes how to move from your typical saturated-fat, fast-food diet to one that sounds so different?

DR. WILLETT BUILDS A NEW PYRAMID

Dr. Walter Willett of the Harvard School of Public Health, a renowned leader in the forefront of medical nutrition, took the healthy eating patterns of the Mediterranean approach to eating and constructed a new food pyramid. Dr. Willett had the scientific integrity to question the federal dietary recommendations, identify the worst and best eating patterns, and build a new food pyramid, one which virtually flipped the old pyramid upside down.

In Dr. Willett's food pyramid, daily exercise and weight control form the foundation of the structure. Next he adds whole-grain foods at most meals along with plant oils, including olive, corn, canola, sunflower, peanut, and other liquid vegetable oils. The next layer of the pyramid contains abundant vegetables and fruits, then daily portions of nuts and legumes. The next layer features healthy sources of protein, including fish, poultry, and eggs. The top layers include dairy or calcium supplements. Red meat, butter, white breads, potatoes, and sweets are at the very top of his pyramid. And, just as it should be, alcohol in moderation is at the side.[55]

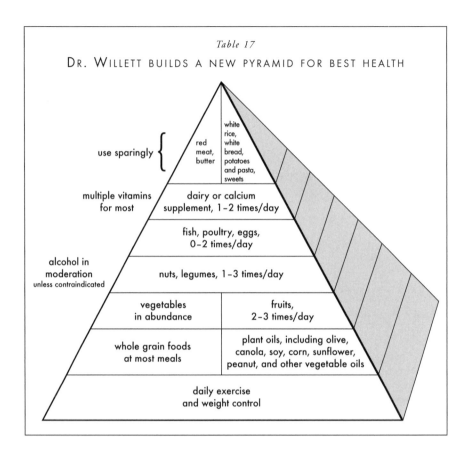

Table 17

DR. WILLETT BUILDS A NEW PYRAMID FOR BEST HEALTH

use sparingly {
red meat, butter | white rice, white bread, potatoes and pasta, sweets

multiple vitamins for most | dairy or calcium supplement, 1–2 times/day

fish, poultry, eggs, 0–2 times/day

alcohol in moderation unless contraindicated | nuts, legumes, 1–3 times/day

vegetables in abundance | fruits, 2–3 times/day

whole grain foods at most meals | plant oils, including olive, canola, soy, corn, sunflower, peanut, and other vegetable oils

daily exercise and weight control

Dr. Willett then went back and studied the health impact of his pyramid. He said, "we found that men and women who were eating in accordance with the new pyramid had a lower risk of major chronic disease. This benefit resulted almost entirely from significant reductions in the risk of cardiovascular disease—up to 30% for women and 40% for men. Following the new pyramid's guidelines did not, however, lower the risk of cancer. Weight control and physical activity, rather than specific food choices, are associated with a reduced risk of many cancers."[56]

THE MEDITERRANEAN DIET IS AN INTERNATIONAL PYRAMID

Many people identify this whole package of healthy eating practices as a Mediterranean diet. The Mediterranean diet is a comprehensive and satisfying way of eating, not a restricted focus on one food or one single part of eating. It is neither low-carb nor low-fat. Rather, it is a whole way of eating health-promoting foods.

This Mediterranean food pyramid can also be built using colorful fruits and vegetables, whole grains, nuts and beans, monounsaturated or polyunsaturated oils, and fish from other cultures. Asian or Indian or African food pyramids can be built with the same components. In the U.S., this Mediterranean pyramid works equally well when adapted to local foods in the deep South, the rural West, the agricultural Midwest, or trendy Manhattan. The diet can be adopted equally by the native born and by immigrants from around the world. The colorful fruit and vegetable, whole-grain, nuts, fish, and olive oil components remain the same but the specific foods and spices vary in keeping with the traditions of various cultures.

A caution: You *can* have too much of a good thing. The Mediterranean diet loses some of its benefits if you push the calories up to traditional American excess. Portion control is an integral part of the success of the Mediterranean way of eating. One difference between the classic Mediterranean plan and the American eating style centers on the total number of calories eaten. In general, our southern European and North African counterparts eat less than we do at any given meal, and they snack much less frequently. We must remember to watch our portion sizes.

EATING AS AN "INFORMED CHOICE"

This multicolored, multispiced, multicountry approach to eating is more a lifelong lifestyle than a diet. It is a broad plan that permits you to choose from a great many foods you like. You should understand the science behind the various parts of this eating plan and why they promote your good health. Once you understand how the foods benefit you, you will be making "Informed Choices."

So here is the basic outline of Informed Choice, my best health-promoting eating plan in its simplest form. The details are explained below:

There are 7 definite steps in my Informed Choice way of eating:

1. Do eat 5 to 7 servings of colorful fruits and vegetables per day.

2. Do eat 2 whole grains per day.

3. Do use liquid monosaturated or polyunsaturated oils.

4. Do eat nuts and legumes (beans) at least twice a week.

5. Do eat fish at least two times a week.

6. Do limit your portion size.

7. Do think about whether the food you are eating has any nutritionally redeeming value.

The Informed Choice Plan is not a diet. Instead, it is a way of approaching food, knowing what foods promote your good health, what foods undermine your good health, and then making an informed decision. The Informed Choice approach focuses on foods that furnish you with nutritional benefits, taste wonderful, and keep you away from craving junk food. The Informed Choice Plan also asks that you limit your intake of empty or harmful foods. By eating the healthy foods listed above, you will automatically decrease the amount of unhealthy food you eat.

Once you start to make Informed Choices you will no longer need to follow fads such as the Atkins or Zone or grapefruit diets. Whether you are trying to be healthy or lose weight, start your new lifetime eating plan by steering away from convenience foods loaded with processed flours and sugars or deep fried foods. Focus on eating portion-controlled sizes of colorful fruits and vegetables, and high-quality protein like fish, eggs, or chicken; or, if you want a red meat, go for the tenderloin. Add high quality carbs in the form of whole-grain cereals or breads. And cook with olive or canola or other liquid oils.

I do not expect or even want you to totally change what you eat by tomorrow morning. You have favorite foods. You have long-standing eating patterns and traditions. You have lunch partners and usual places to go. Plus, you have a whole cupboard of food to use first. But I do want you to start identifying a way of healthy eating you can do for the rest of your life.

So change gradually. As you change, always make an Informed Choice in the direction of better health. Trade up the food scale. Eat a little healthier today than you did yesteday. You have to learn how to make Informed Choices in such a way that you can eat like this forever. The rest of this chapter will give you the information you need to make these choices, discuss why these changes are important, and show you how to get started.

If you want to read more about healthy eating, go to the web site of the Harvard School of Public Health at http://www.hsph.harvard.edu/nutritionsource/index.html. This is an excellent site.

THE IMPORTANCE OF COLORFUL FRUITS AND VEGGIES

Even if you are not ready to adopt the entire Mediterranean diet and can make only one change to your approach to eating right now, begin by adding colorful fruits and vegetables to your diet. Apples, strawberries, broccoli, oranges, sweet potatoes, green beans, beets, spinach, papaya, asparagus, kiwi. Anything colorful. The more colors the better.

Americans eat woefully few fruits and vegetables. The average person eats only one or two colorful fruits and vegetables per day. And almost as bad, we tend to eat the same 10 fruits and vegetables over and over. Our 10 typical fruits and vegetables look something like this: a glass of OJ for breakfast, a salad made with iceberg lettuce, French fries, green beans, or broccoli or corn, and an occasional orange, banana, apple, or bunch of grapes. The tomato as sauce in the pizza also counts. And potatoes.

Sorry. Neither French fries nor iceberg lettuce counts as healthy, colorful vegetables. Granted, technically speaking, iceberg lettuce and potatoes are vegetables. But both these commonly eaten vegetables just happen to be among the lowest in nutrients.

WHAT DOES SCIENCE SAY ABOUT FRUITS AND VEGETABLES?

Science has not yet even identified all of the beneficial chemicals in colorful fruits and vegetables. The more science learns, the more valuable colorful fruits and vegetables become. They contain hundreds of highly protective phytochemicals (phyto = plant, i.e., plant chemicals), vitamins, and antioxidants that proactively lower heart disease and cancer. You cannot find these benefits in a pill. An array of colorful fruits and vegetables gives you an all-you-need variety of phytochemicals, antioxidants, and vitamins.

Every health study sends the same message, loud and clear: eating a wide variety of colorful fruits and vegetables reduces disease and promotes health.

> *Note: As a careful reader, you will note some inconsistencies in the scientific numbers quoted in this section. Outcomes will vary slightly because researchers cannot control all of the differences in foods and people. The important lesson to take home is that all of the studies confirm the benefits of eating the Informed Choice Plan.*

The key idea here is *wide variety of colors*. A broad color palette ensures that you get all of the different health-promoting chemicals. Red beets, orange squash, purple plums, green broccoli, and pink grapefruit. The more colors and the wider the variety of types of fruits and veggies you eat every week, the more healthy the total package.

◆ The Physicians' Health Study and the Nurses' Health Study monitored more than 100,000 people. The people who ate the most fruits and vegetables experienced 20% less heart disease than the people who ate the least. Researchers further calculated that each daily serving of colorful fruits and vegetables reduced the risk of heart disease by 4%.[57]

◆ Fruits and vegetables fight obesity. Eating meals with added vegetables in place of added starches can reduce your total calorie intake by 20% to 30%.[58]

◆ The National Weight Control Registry studies people who have lost more than 30 pounds and kept the weight off for more than a year. These successful dieters had three things in common: they ate fewer calories, they ate more fruits and vegetables, and they exercised.[59]

◆ The European EPIC Study reported that eating one pound of fruits and vegetables per day reduced the risk of cancer of the upper digestive tract by 50%.[60]

◆ Multiple studies report that eating fruits and vegetables, particularly tomatoes and the veggies in the broccoli family, reduces cancer.

◆ A Danish study estimated that by doubling the daily fruit and vegetable intake, the average person would decrease their risk of cancer by 19% to 32%.[61]

Taken together, these studies more than confirm that a diet which includes five or more colorful fruits and vegetables per day reduces heart disease, cancer, obesity, and diabetes.

Where to Start

You need at least five servings of colorful fruits and vegetables every day. Blueberries, green spinach, red tomatoes, orange mangoes, yellow peppers all have different health-promoting phytochemicals. Fruits and veggies can enhance and brighten any meal or snack. Fortunately, Mother Nature has prepackaged many fruits and vegetables for easy travel and eating on the run.

Count them. Start your day with a glass of (1) OJ and (2) berries on your whole grain cereal. Lunch is pasta with (3) tomato sauce, and for dessert an (4) orange. Your afternoon snack? (5) Grapes have as much sugar and sweetness as a candy bar but none of the bad fats or processed chemicals. Put your sautéed chicken breast on a bed of (6) bright spinach and (7) mushrooms. Enjoy a (8) sweet potato. Fabulous. You can include a (9) peach cobbler for dessert—just don't eat the crust. And you didn't think you could add five fruits and veggies a day?

Some might argue that fresh fruits and veggies are too expensive. To minimize cost, buy in season or buy frozen, as long as the frozen kind do not contain added sugars or high-fructose corn syrup.

The Importance of Whole Grains

The following are carbohydrates: whole wheat, oatmeal, white flour, potatoes, and sugar. They appear in the food we eat as whole-wheat bread, hot oatmeal, spaghetti, mashed potatoes, and the sugar we add to our tea. Carbohydrates are sugars of varying lengths strung together. There are good carbs and bad carbs. And now, apparently, "net carbs." Be careful—a net carb is more an advertising gimmick than a food group.

Here's the problem. What starts life as a perfectly good carbo-hydrate, whole wheat, is most often highly processed into nutri-tionally poor white flour and made into white breads, cookies, crackers, and cereals. This refined and processed flour is readily absorbed as a simple sugar without much other nutritive value.

The whole-wheat kernel has three parts: the germ, which con-tains the very healthy oils; the bran, which contains the fiber; and the endosperm, which contains the carbohydrate. All good things but best eaten as one combined package. After whole wheat is "refined" into white flour, only the carbohydrate-dense starch—the sugar—remains. The germ and the bran are gone. The pro-cessing may remove 70% to 90% of the vitamins and minerals from the original whole wheat. And then, because the refiner removed all of the healthy parts of the wheat germ, the refiner "enriches" the flour by adding back vitamins and some minerals.

The result is that your breakfast bagel is not much different than a bowl of sugar to your body biochemistry. Eat a bagel for breakfast or pretzels for a snack, and your body quickly breaks down the simple flour molecules and absorbs them as sugar mole-cules. Your blood sugar spikes, insulin rises, blood sugar falls, and two hours later, you are hungry again.

No-carb diets work because they stop this cycle. They move you away from the nutritionally poor processed flours like bagels, pretzels, chips, and cookies that you absorb so quickly. The low-carb replacements of protein and fat are, by comparison, much more slowly absorbed from your stomach.

Whole-wheat flour, on the other hand, contains the entire wheat kernel, all three parts, ground together as a whole. Whole-wheat flour contains all of the nutrients in the germ, the bran, and the endosperm. Nothing is removed. When you eat whole-wheat toast, not only do you get the nutritional value of the wheat germ, but the fiber of the bran slows the carbohydrate absorption.

When you choose to eat whole-grain bread, rather than nutritionally emptier white bread, your entire biochemistry process reacts differently. The whole grain is digested much more slowly, the sugars in the carbohydrates are absorbed more slowly, your blood sugar rises more slowly, and your insulin level rises more slowly and to lower peaks. You will not be hungry 90 minutes later because your blood sugars do not spike and then crash. In addition, you also benefit from the nutrients in the germ and the fiber in the bran.

WHAT DOES SCIENCE SAY ABOUT WHOLE GRAINS?

- ◆ Again, the Nurses' Health Study sheds light on the health benefits of eating whole grains. The study of nearly 72,000 women showed that those with the highest intake of cereal fiber dropped their risk of heart disease by one-third, compared to the group that ate the least cereal fiber.[62]

- ◆ In the Physicians' Health Study of 86,000 men, about 20% of the men reported eating one bowl of cereal per day, and about 10% reported eating one bowl of whole-grain cereal per day. The men who ate the bowl of whole-grain cereal per day showed a 27% reduction in heart disease. However, eating cereals made from processed wheat had no impact on heart disease.[63]

- ◆ The health of these men benefited from as little as one serving of whole grains (measured as five grams of fiber) per day, but the best results show themselves at two or three whole-grain servings. How much is that? A bowl of oatmeal or Total and a slice of whole-wheat bread for breakfast. Eating one or two or three whole grains a day will substantially reduce your risk of heart disease, cancer, and diabetes.

Buying Good Bread Is Harder than You Think

When you shop for bread, you should read the fine print on the labels—don't take the words such as "wheat bread" on the big label at face value. You are looking for bread with a label that lists "ground whole wheat" as the first ingredient (ingredients are listed in descending order of use in the product.)

Breads whose ingredient labels use phrases like "enriched wheat," "refined whole wheat," "seven grain," or "oatmeal bread" are not whole-grain products. Beware: all of these phrases tell you that the manufacturer has taken processed white flour, "enriched" it by adding back some of the nutrients taken out during processing, added a little bit of molasses as food color, and given the bread a healthy-sounding name. Voilà, plain white bread has been made to look and sound nutritious.

Where to Start Making Carbohydrates Healthy?

You need all three parts of whole grain to receive its full nutritive value. A diet of white flour and bran cereal omits the germ, which contains the greatest concentration of nutrients.

◆ Breakfast cereals are one of the most widely available sources of whole grains. Shredded wheat and oatmeal are two wonderful and easy examples.

◆ You'll find several varieties of whole-grain bread on the market, and many of them taste wonderful.

◆ Other sources of whole grain? Have barley soup for lunch. Make a salad with bulgur and corn and tomatoes. Cook some bulgur pilaf with dried apricots, dates, and pine nuts. Explore two little-known grains, quinoa and amaranth, which you can find in the health food aisle in larger grocery stores.

◆ Balance your carbs. You have to eat your whole grains as a breakfast cereal or as whole-wheat toast because you'll never see an angel food cake made from whole wheat. Nor should you expect to. Grains have different uses. Shredded wheat for breakfast, whole-grain bread for lunch, and quinoa pilaf at dinner. Get your grain nutrients throughout the day, so you can enjoy all the glory of the chocolate sponge cake made with refined cake flour as a dessert treat.

THE IMPORTANCE OF USING HEALTHY OILS

The *kind of fat* you eat is far more important than *the amount of fat* you eat. Some fats actually promote good health, while other fats are lethal, hastening heart disease, diabetes, and some cancers.

Bad fats, including both saturated and trans fats, are solid at room temperature—and equally solid inside your arteries, where they cause heart attacks. The truth is that Americans eat huge amounts of food that contain saturated and trans fats. Large amounts of "bad fat" are a major cause of our high rates of cancer and heart disease.

Health-promoting oils, including the monounsaturated or polyunsaturated oils, are liquid at room temperature. These oils may actually promote good health with a lower risk of cancer, heart disease, and diabetes as we shall see in a few pages.

America today seems obsessed with either a low-fat diet or the Atkins high-fat diet. Let's look at the facts about fats and oils:

◆ No study has ever shown that a low-fat diet has health benefits.[64] A low-fat diet is good for your health only because it moves you away from the bad saturated and trans fats.

◆ Hundreds of studies document the ill health caused by eating foods high in saturated fat and the harm caused by trans-fatty acids.

◆ Numerous studies show the benefits of a diet that contains healthy fats and avoids unhealthy fats.

◆ The type of fat eaten matters much more than the quantity of fat. Table 18 shows that even though the population studied in Crete got 40% of their calories from monounsaturated fats (olive oils), this group has the lowest number of deaths from heart attacks. The population of Japan gets a mere 10% of their calories from fat, about as low as you can go, yet their death rate from heart disease exceeds that of Crete. And Finland gets 40% of their total calories from saturated fats (butter), and they post the highest death rate from heart disease in the study group. The moral seems clear and consistent with other studies: a diet high in unhealthy fats is bad for you while a diet high in healthy oils is good for you.

		Japan	Finland	Crete
Table 18 RATES OF HEART DISEASE COMPARED TO FAT CONSUMPTION Source: Walter C. Willett and Meir J. Stampfer, "Rebuilding the Food Pyramid," Scientific American (Jan. 2003):65–71 (modified).				
% of daily calories from fat		10%	38%	40%
Predominant type of fat in diet		All fat	Saturated fat	Olive oil
Rates of coronary artery disease per 10,000 men over 10 years		500	3,000	200

Watching your fat intake when practicing the Informed Choice eating plan is as simple as knowing there are good and bad fats and oils. We should enjoy the good and healthy fats in moderation, and we should avoid the bad fats.

THE TRANS-FAT TRAP

Trans-fatty acids may well be the worst fats for your health. You'll find them listed on labels as "partially hydrogenated" fats and oils. These fats are hidden from you as ingredients in the prepared or deep-fried foods you eat. Manufacturers use trans fats because they are cheap, easy to work with, and prolong the shelf life of products. A partially hydrogenated soybean oil is as bad for you as partially hydrogenated coconut oil. Manufacturers may call these trans fats "margarine" or "shortening." Do not be fooled. These trans fats both raise your bad cholesterol and lower your good cholesterol.

How do you recognize a trans fat? Right now, the only way to find trans fats is to read labels, looking for the words "partially hydrogenated." The government will require manufacturers to list the grams of trans fats on packages soon. Or you can go to www.cpsinet.org for a list of trans fats in foods, or you can look for the words "hydrogenated," "partially hydrogenated," or "shortening" on a food label. Never eat foods with a trans fat near the top of an ingredient list. You are probably okay if "partially hydrogenated" appears near the bottom of the ingredient list because ingredients are listed in descending order according to the amounts the product contains.

MORE SCIENCE ON TRANS FATS

Women who eat the most trans fats are almost 50% more likely to develop heart disease than women who eat the least trans fats.[65] Prepared foods are often made with trans fats. The women who ate the most trans fats ate about 3% of their daily calories as trans fats. If a woman eats 2,000 calories per day, then 3% is 60 calories per day or about a teaspoon and a half of trans fats per day. Want to know what a teaspoon and a half of trans fats look like? One and a half doughnuts, a large size order of fast-food fries, or 36 Ritz crackers. There is a silver lining in every cloud: now that you know about trans fats, you can halve your risk of heart disease by identifying and avoiding them.

HOW TO START TO EAT HEALTHIER FATS AND OILS

◆ Read labels. Immediately reduce your intake of trans-fatty acids to as little as possible. This means no doughnuts, fried foods, and most bakery goods.

◆ Start to reduce your intake of saturated fats. This means eating less red meat, or when you eat red meat, always go for a leaner cut of meat. No more rib-eye steak, but you can say yes to tenderloin.

◆ Use monounsaturated oils such as olive or canola oil whenever possible. Alternatively, use the liquid polyunsaturated oils such as corn or soybean. Use these oils for cooking, as a salad dressing, and on vegetables.

THE IMPORTANCE OF NUTS AND LEGUMES

Nuts have gone from banned as "bad for you" to nutrition's front row. Nuts are a great example of how even small amounts of certain foods can have a very positive impact on your health. True, nuts get 80% of their calories from fat. But the fat is primarily a monounsaturated, very-good-for-your-health fat.

The first clue that nuts promote good health came from the health study of 30,000 Seventh Day Adventists. To the researcher's surprise, people who reported eating nuts had a lower risk of heart disease. People who ate nuts daily had a 50% lower risk of heart disease than those who did not eat nuts at all. Even a small handful of nuts once or twice a week is beneficial.[66]

Other studies have shown nuts can lower cholesterol. But the improvement in heart risk is greater than just lower cholesterol. The kind of nut does not appear to matter. So please enjoy a small handful of almonds, walnuts, pecans, macadamias, hazelnuts, or Brazil nuts a couple of times per week.

THE IMPORTANCE OF FISH

You should eat fish, preferably saltwater fish, regularly. Fish contain two essential fatty acids, omega-3 and omega-6. Even though these fats are essential for good cellular functioning, the human body cannot make them. These compounds, particularly omega-3, reduce inflammation in cells and reduce blood-clotting tendencies. Cellular inflammation and increased clotting are major causes of blood vessel damage and disease. Eating fish high in omega-3 has also been linked to stabilizing heart rhythms and reducing high triglycerides, which also reduces the risk of heart disease. Omega-3 is also necessary for normal brain functioning.

There is considerable debate about which fish contains how much omega-3. The amount of omega-3 in a fish depends on whether the fish is farm-raised or wild, what the fish ate, and the season of the year in which it was harvested. In general, salmon, sardines, bluefish, rainbow trout, and striped bass all have much higher levels of omega-3 than catfish or lobster, which have almost none.

Having said that, eating fish is almost always better than eating red meat. Fish does not contain saturated fats, unless it was fried in these fats. A study published in the *New England Journal of Medicine*[67] reported that people who ate fish twice a week showed a 50% lower rate of fatal heart attacks than those who did not eat fish. This is an astonishingly powerful statement.

WHERE TO START

- ◆ Eat fish at least twice a week. If you don't eat much fish now, begin to experiment. Many more kinds of fish are available in the supermarket than ever before. Salmon, tuna, swordfish, shark, mahi-mahi, sardines, bluefish, rainbow trout, striped bass, and mackerel. Aim for saltwater fish which are much higher in the valuable omega-3's than freshwater fish.

◆ Make an Informed Choice about preparing fish. Don't roll them in flour and bread them. Don't deep-fat fry them. Steam, grill, microwave, or sauté them in olive oil.

HOW TO START THE INFORMED CHOICE EATING PLAN

◆ **Use fresh ingredients.** The easiest way to change your eating habits is to start with fresh ingredients. This also guarantees more colorful fruits and vegetables.

The hardest meals to change are those that start with already prepared convenience foods. Any recipe that starts with a can of cream of mushroom soup, a cup of sour cream, or several tablespoons of mayonnaise is almost beyond salvation. Best to throw that recipe out and look for one where you control the ingredients. You just cannot make a cheesecake recipe containing cream cheese and sour cream into a healthy Informed Choice–approved food. Instead, make a fruit tart. If you can't buy a pizza without heavy cheese and sausage, make your own. My bakery sells pizza dough that I roll out, paint with olive oil, cover with diced tomatoes, artichokes, Canadian bacon (it's a lot less fatty than sausage), and a liberal sprinkling of Parmesan cheese. Use everything you've learned about foods in this chapter to create your own version of the Informed Choice Plan.

◆ **Lose weight.** If you're trying to lose weight as well as change your eating style, understand that this plan works as a diet only if you also follow all of the exercise and portion control prescriptions above. Remember, weight is a balance of calories in and calories out. You must exercise—walk if nothing else—to increase the number of calories you burn.

◆ **Think before you buy groceries.** If the only things you have in the house for snacking are a bag of chips and a bag of cookies, you have a little farther to go to get to the starting line. You either have to look harder in the cupboard or rethink what you keep in your cupboard and refrigerator. You are aiming for a more healthy array of foods. Buy nuts instead of chips. Buy granola bars instead of cookies. Make a berry pie instead of buying store-made frosted brownies.

◆ **Move slowly to make the plan work.** Always trade up for health. Day by day, try to pass up an unhealthy food and choose a slightly more healthy food. This keeps you eating foods you like, just always choosing the slightly more healthy option. You might not be able to move from store-bought cookies to an apple right away. But you can move from the cellophane-wrapped cookie made with trans-fatty acids, highly refined wheat, and sugar to a chocolate bar with nuts (which contains only chocolate and nuts). At least you just got rid of the partially hydrogenated oils and white flour. Hey, it's a step in the right direction.

Charlie trades up.

Charlie started to think about food more carefully after he watched a public television show on nutrition. While the

PBS show had nudged him toward making slightly healthier choices, he told himself that he was never going to "get carried away" to extremes. No tofu burgers or bean sprouts for him.

Charlie, to his surprise, found that making informed choices was not all that difficult. He found that he did have choices that all worked with foods and tastes he liked.

Some of his choices were easy. A bowl of Wheaties (whole grain) instead of Fruit Loops. A tuna salad sandwich instead of a cheeseburger. A diet soda instead of a shake. Large fries became small fries, and eventually no fries. A large steak became a medium steak, became a tenderloin, and then a piece of salmon (that complete change took over a year).

◆ **Read labels when you shop.** The grocery store offers you choices. If you need crackers, you have lots to choose from. Read the labels until you find something, like Ak-Mak crackers, which lists ingredients as "100% stone-ground whole-of-the-wheat flour, water, clover honey, sesame oil, dairy butter, sesame seeds, yeast and salt."

◆ **Choose good proteins.** When you need meat, choose deep-water fish instead of catfish; choose the leanest ground meat or the flank steak instead of the rib-eye steak. A poached egg on whole wheat toast is a much better start to the day than pancakes with syrup.

◆ **Trade up the health food ladder.** At a buffet or party, choose the nuts over the chips; choose fruit over cheese. At a restaurant, choose a spinach salad instead of iceberg lettuce. Trade from heart-damaging trans-fatty-acid chips to heart-healthy nuts. Yes, you can have popcorn at the movies—just order a small size. Medium size if you are going to share it. Yes, you can go to a fast-food restaurant; just stick with a single hamburger and don't super-size it. Yes, you can eat pizza—just not the double-cheese one. Yes, you can eat dessert, just not all of it, or order a fruit cobbler instead of the chocolate torte.

◆ **Is this always?** Does this mean you can never have a steak again? No. You can still have New York strip steak, just much less often. Eat about half of it, and save the rest for another day.

Summary and Checklist

Changing your eating plan not only means doing the right thing. It also means no longer doing the wrong thing. Here are two lists for you:

The Absolute "Do Not" List

1. Do not eat anything called "super-size" or "jumbo."

2. Do not eat "double" anything. That includes double-bacon cheeseburger, double-cheese pizza, double-thick malts, double cocktails at Happy Hour.

3. Do not eat junk food until the manufacturers start to make healthy junk food.

4. Do not eat highly processed prepared foods unless you have read the label to know they are prepared with your heart in mind.

5. Do not eat fried foods.

6. Do not eat from the bag or carton.

The Absolute "Do" List

1. Know and eat the right portion size.

2. Choose and eat health-promoting, disease-fighting foods.

3. Eat at least five to seven colorful fruits and veggie portions per day.

4. Eat two whole-grain portions per day.

5. Eat fish twice a week.

6. Eat nuts at least twice a week.

7. Cook with monounsaturated or polyunsaturated (liquid) oils only.

The goal of this Informed Choice eating plan is to eat normal portions of health-promoting food in place of larger portions of harmful food. The goal is to find and keep changes to your eating plan that enable you to stick with this new way of eating tomorrow, the next day, the day after that, and forever.

Dr. Bob's promise:

◆ *Your body will thank you for this change.*

Take a look at Charlie now, one year later.

Charlie has slowly come to better understand what he should eat. Now he thinks before he eats.

When he makes breakfast for himself and the kids, he fixes sliced melon, shredded wheat with strawberries, or a fruit smoothie made with yogurt and bananas, orange juice, and whatever fruits are in the fridge or freezer. Sometimes it's scrambled eggs with whole-wheat toast and jam. And coffee.

Interestingly, Charlie has found he is seldom hungry in the morning and does not need a morning snack.

Lunch is often a piece of fish or grilled chicken breast on a dark green lettuce salad served with olive oil and vinegar. During the winter, he loves to eat chili or white bean soups. Dessert is an orange or apple or big bunch of grapes. It has taken Charlie considerable effort to persuade the restaurant to add fresh fruit to the dessert menu, but it has turned out to be a big seller.

At four o'clock, he still gets hungry. He keeps a jar of nuts and trail mix in his desk drawer. He finds that if he munches a handful, he's good for the rest of the day.

For dinner, Charlie still has trouble because of the kids' after-school activities. But he and his wife both make certain that the house has a lot more nuts and whole-grain crackers for snacking. Dinner is more chicken and tuna— and less beef. And always, dinner now includes something like a sweet potato and broccoli or grilled asparagus. He has even taken to cooking the broccoli Italian-style with raisins and pine nuts. Awesome. Gone are the hot dogs and potato chips. Dessert has became distinctly less frequent, but on dessert nights, the family enjoys baked peaches.

Without much effort over the course of a year, Charlie began to lose weight. He loved what he was eating, and he was not as hungry as before. Charlie knew he was onto something good.

Make Informed Choices. Simple choices, big changes. Avoid disease-promoting foods. Choose health-promoting foods and smaller portions. Reduce the risk of cancer, protect your blood vessels. Lower the risk of heart disease and stroke. Control your future health. That's the plan. Think of this as your "plan for life."

Chapter 8

ALCOHOL: A TOAST
TO YOUR HEART

Drinking alcohol is a complex issue, surrounded by social graces, safety concerns, religious prohibitions, health benefits, and health cautions—all poured into one glass. The health effects of alcohol range from clearly beneficial to clearly fatal.

It's all a matter of degree. Multiple large health studies show that people who drink small to moderate amounts of alcohol live healthier lives than either nondrinkers or heavy drinkers. In fact, drinking small to moderate amounts of alcohol may be more healthy than not drinking at all. But drinking too much is worse than not drinking at all. And if you do not drink, none of these studies should persuade you to start.

Who drinks in America—and how much?

- More than 30% of adult Americans do not drink alcohol at all or have fewer than 12 drinks per year.

- About 50%–60% of adults drink alcohol responsibly and moderately.

◆ The remaining 10% of adults drink about half of all alcohol poured in America.

WHAT IS A DRINK?

To an American researcher, a "drink" is defined as 15 cc of ethanol, about one-half ounce of alcohol, which just happens to be the amount of alcohol in a standard 12-ounce bottle of beer; or 1.5 ounces of gin, vodka, bourbon, or scotch; or 5 ounces of wine.

While the federal government and alcohol researchers have a clear definition of a drink, this definition often falls apart in real life. Determining how much alcohol is in your drink is not easy, even if you are sober.

◆ Most beers contain about 4.5% to 5.5% alcohol. Light beers are about 3.0% to 4.5% alcohol. But some specialty beers contain upward of 8.5% alcohol.

◆ Most white wine is about 11% alcohol; most reds are about 13%.

◆ Fortified wines, such as sherry, port, and Madeira range from 17% to 20% alcohol.

◆ And hard liquor can fall anywhere from 35% to 50% alcohol, expressed as *proof* on the bottle. The proof is twice the percent of ethanol in the bottle. An 86-proof gin contains 43% alcohol.

To add another layer of complexity to the measuring process, there's the problem of defining "a drink" served in a bar or restaurant. Just as food portions have gotten larger, so too have alcohol portions. One drink in a restaurant before dinner is often much larger than one drink defined by a researcher.

◆ Today's restaurant-made martini is anywhere between 1.5 and 4.5 ounces of vodka. That makes the cocktail-hour martini equal to anywhere from one to three standard drinks.

◆ A mixed drink can also vary in size from 1.5 ounces to 5 ounces. The recipe for a Long Island Iced Tea calls for five 40-proof alcohols (vodka, gin, tequila, rum, and triple sec) and a splash of Coca Cola. A standard size drink, then, would require no more than 1 teaspoon of each ingredient. An unlikely event.

If you have dinner after the cocktail hour, you might add a bottle of wine to your evening. And that is how you slide right past the legal blood-alcohol limit of 0.8 to drive. If you drink like this anywhere other than your own kitchen, please get a ride home.

WHO DRINKS HOW MUCH?

The National Institute of Alcohol Abuse and Alcoholism (NIAAA) keeps numbers on alcohol consumption in America. The chart below shows who drinks how much.

	Table 19 — The NIAAA Definitions of Who Drinks How Much in America				
	Lifetime abstainer	Former drinker	Light drinker	Moderate drinker	Heavy drinker
	Fewer than 12 drinks per year	None	More than 12 drinks per year but fewer than 3 drinks per week	3 to 14 drinks per week	More than 2 drinks per day on average
% of both sexes	34%	22	19	17	7
Men (%)	22	23	21	23	12
Women (%)	45	21	18	12	3

A Drink a Day Does Not Mean an Ice Tea Tumbler

Heavy drinking is common in America. The NIAAA 2004 statistics estimate that 7% to 8% of adults in this country—20 million Americans—abuse alcohol or have a dependency problem (4.5% abuse alcohol and 3.8% are alcoholic.).[68]

The NIAAA study defines alcohol abuse as causing a failure to fulfill major role obligations at work, school, or home; creating interpersonal, social, and legal problems; and/or drinking in hazardous situations. Alcohol dependence, also known as alcoholism, is characterized by impaired control over drinking, compulsive drinking, preoccupation with drinking, tolerance to alcohol, and/or withdrawal symptoms.

We all know that heavy or out-of-control drinking is dangerous and harmful—causing heart disease, liver disease, cancer, accidents, trauma, violence, homicide, and suicide. Heavy drinking interferes with work, social obligations, and family life.

Alcohol is linked with 100,000 deaths each year:

◆ 40% of all auto accidents are drink-related.

◆ 10,000 deaths each year are the result of alcohol-induced cirrhosis of the liver. Who is at-risk in this widely quoted statistic? People who consistently drink 80 grams of ethanol per day: that's eight standard beers, a bottle of wine, or five shots of hard liquor.

As the ancient Chinese saying goes: First the man has a drink. Then the drink has a drink. Then the drink has the man.

Let's congratulate the people who have acknowledged that they have a problem controlling alcohol or that alcohol controls them. It's a very difficult and personal insight. But amazingly, if this poor health habit is corrected, just as with any other of the habits discussed in this book, the body can recover and repair. These people can continue to gain health benefits by following all of the other recommendations: don't smoke, maintain normal weight, exercise 30 minutes most days of the week, and eat a diet high in fruits and vegetables.

WHAT IS DRINKING IN MODERATION?

As table 19 shows, drinking moderately means consuming anywhere from 3 to 14 drinks a week. The truth is that the health benefits of alcohol start with drinking as little as a glass of wine (or any other drink) once a week. For the majority of people, moderate drinking means social drinking at meals or with friends and is not associated with health problems. The health risks of alcohol begin to exceed the health benefits at more than three drinks per day. Note: In general, because a woman has a lesser ability to metabolize alcohol, a woman's safe limit is 25% lower than a man's.

HEALTH BENEFITS FOR THOSE WHO DRINK ALCOHOL MODERATELY

Multiple studies have documented clearly and consistently the health benefits of low-to-moderate alcohol consumption when compared to abstinence or heavy drinking. Almost all of the benefits of alcohol center on reducing cardiovascular risk, specifically heart attacks, strokes, and peripheral arterial disease. The people who benefited most were those who drank one drink every other day to two drinks per day.

And the benefit was quite substantial: reducing the risk of heart disease by about 30%.[69] The benefit in women was offset by a slight increase in the risk of breast cancer among women who had two or more drinks per day.[70]

Studies all show that when plotted on a graph, the benefits of alcohol consumption form a U shape. The greatest benefit occurs with occasional to moderate drinking—the low point in the U, while both abstainers and abusers, the legs of the U, are at higher risk than light to moderate drinkers. This statement is supported by research from the Honolulu Heart Study, the Physicians' Health Study, and the British Physicians' Study. The National Institute on Alcohol Abuse and Alcoholism states, "The totality of evidence on moderate alcohol and [heart disease] supports a judgment of a cause-effect relationship...there are cardio-protective benefits associated with responsible moderate alcohol intake."[71]

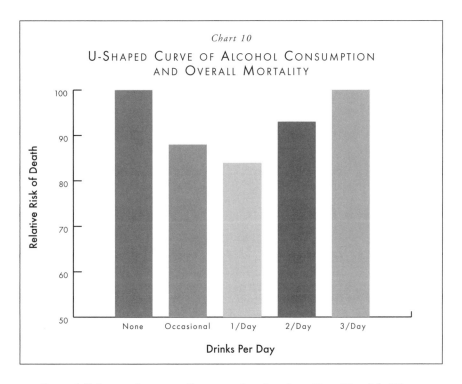

Chart 10
U-SHAPED CURVE OF ALCOHOL CONSUMPTION
AND OVERALL MORTALITY

In addition, the excellent web site by Dr. David Hanson, http://www2.potsdam.edu/alcohol-info/AlcoholAndHealth.html, reports on studies totaling more than 400,000 people. These studies consistently demonstrate that:

◆ moderate drinkers experience lower death rate than non-drinkers or heavy drinkers;

◆ moderate drinkers develop less disability than the general population; and

◆ moderate drinking lowers the risk of heart attack by 30%.

While no one can adequately explain the mechanism by which alcohol reduces mortality, most scientists agree that alcohol reduces blood clotting, reduces blood pressure, and improves the blood cholesterol profile by raising the good HDL cholesterol.

A drink or two for men and one a day for women seem to provide real health benefits. It does not matter if the beverage is wine or gin or beer. Yet the health effect of red wine appears stronger than other alcohols. The oft-cited "French paradox" is the low death rate among the Gallic crowd, despite diets high in butter, rich meats, and cheese. While the French consume about the same amount of alcohol as other populations, some researchers speculate that an antioxidant in red wine is responsible for France's better life expectancy.

Dr. Bob recommends:

◆ *If you cannot control your drinking, you are clearly better off not drinking at all.*

◆ *If you find drinking unacceptable, then sit quietly on the sideline and let this health habit roll past you—which makes all of the other six health recommendations even more important to you.*

◆ *If you drink socially and moderately, take comfort that you are substantially reducing your risk of heart disease.*

◆ *If you drink, enjoy your glass of wine with a Mediterranean dinner shared with good friends. Santé!*

Chapter 9

BE KIND, UNWIND

So, how stressed are you? Can you remember what it is like to be happy? Do you have the time to savor your happiness? Are you in control of your own life? Is there a sense of calm or peace or time just for you somewhere in your hectic day?

Or are you juggling a multitasked life dealing with a demanding boss, a difficult client, an overdue report, after-school soccer games and piano lessons, your e-mail, Palm Pilot, cell phone, and, whoa, the car is leaking oil?

Most of us look upon stress as a part of modern life. And as life grows ever more fast-paced, conveniences like e-mail, pagers, and cell phones only seem to demand more of us, increasing our stress. The pace and competitive pressures of business are skyrocketing. The demands on working mothers and fathers are immense even with good support from a partner. The kids are stressed.

It's a fact: chronic stress damages your health. Yet there are some stresses you can control, reducing their effect or eliminating them. When you cannot control other things that create your stress, you can choose how you react.

In this chapter, I want you to think about stress and its impact on you. Take the short quiz below to see the role stress plays in your life. After you've taken the quiz and learned about your stress level, we'll take a look at the health consequences of stress. And last, we'll talk about how to identify the stressors in your life and manage them.

Self-assessment 3 WHAT'S YOUR STRESS LEVEL?			
How do you feel on most days?	I feel frazzled and overwhelmed.	I am busy, and I have slightly more on my plate than I want.	I am generally happy, calm, and in control.
How is your day job?	I work for and with shortsighted and selfish idiots who harangue me to death every day.	It's not great, but a steady paycheck is important to me.	I love going to work!
How is your money situation?	I am always a dollar short and a payment behind.	I sometimes overspend, but generally I live within my means.	I live within my means and save or invest regularly.
How does anger affect your daily life?	Many situations make me angry—all day long. This anger simmers inside me for hours.	I get angry only sometimes. My anger is short-lived.	I rarely get angry.
Do you make quiet time for yourself?	When would I have time for myself?	I spend time on hobbies or recreation regularly.	I make quiet time for myself. I meditate or take a quiet walk every day.
How closely are you electronically attached to the world?	I carry a cell phone, pager, and PDA at all times.	I am able and willing to turn off my cell, etc., when I want or need to.	After the workday, I limit electronic connections to a couple of hours a day.
Do you multitask?	I can drive, talk on my cell phone, read e-mail, and eat lunch all at the same time.	I check voice mail or e-mail hourly.	I always focus on the task at hand and try to shut out distractions.
How is your social life?	I have few friends.	I have friends, but I do not socialize on a regular basis.	I make time for and give energy to friends and family each week.
Do you consider yourself	Very stressed and in need of stress relief.	Probably average, which means more stress than is good for me.	Unstressed or able to handle stress well.

WHAT IS STRESS?

We all understand stress, but we have trouble putting it into words. Stress is our feeling of being overwhelmed—we feel powerless to control an event or situation, or a series of events or situations. The biggest cause of stress in most of us? Being responsible for getting a task done but lacking the authority, the ability, or the time to do the job or do it well. You were asked to do the task. You *want* to do the task, but there are obstacles that get in your way.

Some stressors are external: a difficult coworker, a report you dread to write, a crisis in your neighborhood, a flooded basement, an ill child, or an increasingly dependent parent.

Other stressors are internal. They can grow out of the pressure we put on ourselves, out of the anger we keep inside, or out of the feelings that boil up in us but are never released.

What's more, stress can feed on itself and cause us to raise our responses a notch. We become more sensitive, angrier, more argumentative—and less tolerant, less supportive, less confident in our abilities, and generally, less in control. All of these characteristics worsen and perpetuate our stress, undermining the very relationships we need to help us get through stressful times.

DAILY STRESSORS

The increased pace and demands of today's frenetic life create anxiety in us all: children and teenagers, young parents, middleaged workers, women returning to the workplace, and retirees. Everyone has stress, some more than others. Consider the contributing factors:

The pace of life. Daily life is a complex blend of scheduled activity, errands, chores, demands from others, the need to race against the clock, and concerns about business and money. There is noise, multiple priorities, and bustle all around us all the time. Most of us hold our lives together only by our supreme effort.

Worries close at hand and far away. We worry about job reviews, succeeding in general, report cards, teenage behavior, drunk drivers, and HIV. The nightly news describes a world on the verge of war, famine, disaster, and one more instance of political or economic chicanery. Religion, once the bastion of stability in our life, has become the focus of divisive internal political arguments and geopolitical conflict. We can control little of it.

To be in the know. We feel constant pressure just to stay connected to everyone else and to follow the news. Think about our grandparents' news cycle. Reports from World War II took hours to travel from the battlefield to a radio office in London and then on to America, where it was set in type for the next edition. Our grandparents read the daily newspaper and listened to some news on the radio. Sometime in the mid-1950s, television evening news shows appeared. Even then, newscasters such as Walter Cronkite were more like everyone's favorite uncle. They delivered the news as carefully condensed stories, complete with background information, and all woven into a meaningful report.

Contrast that with today. The news is always on. The latest war scene or disastrous fire is instantly reported live with minimal background but with close-ups of the calamity. Every car accident or local tragedy enters our living rooms and is replayed every 15 minutes. News of business layoffs are delivered with the ominous implication that we could be next, followed by a story about the possible economic ill effects of more jobless Americans. Medical advances are released before the medical community can agree on the real value of the "breakthrough." Every crime carries with it the threat that it could happen to us if we're not careful. Even our weather is often breathlessly reported as a looming disaster. In short, everything is reported with drama and a sense of urgency. Your personal stress, the result of your day, is heightened by the tension created by such ominous chatter. Bad news becomes the background noise of daily life.

Now add the intrusions of ringing, buzzing, and vibrating of cell phones, pagers, and PDAs—24/7. We are never alone. It's not very different from a criminal who wears an electronic bracelet so that the police can keep tabs on his or her whereabouts. When do you have time to daydream if every quiet moment can be shattered by the ringing of your cell phone?

Structure and competition. Even our own athletics and sports, which could help people release stress, often are valued only if we win. Today's hurried children may never know the fun of a pickup game of baseball or basketball. They know only the stress of organized team sports: with uniforms, coaches, and schedules.

WHY STRESS IS HARMFUL

Measuring the harmful effect of stress is much more difficult than, say, measuring the effect of cigarette smoke. The major problem lies in distinguishing the "bad" parts of stress from the "good" parts of stress. Good stress may motivate you, spur you to produce a better product or reach a higher goal. Another problem? Stress varies from person to person. What stresses one person only moderately may stress another significantly. We all react differently.

Despite our differences, we all experience stress, and we should be concerned with the bad effects of long-term stress on our health. Just as the effects of other lifestyle habits, such as being inactive or overeating, can accumulate over the years and damage your health, so can the effects of stress.

Stress causes the body to release fight-or-flight hormones which speed up your heart and tense your body to prepare for battle or escape. Our ancestors knew this stress as the rare "Uh-oh, there is a big bear outside the cave." By contrast, our stressors are more like to occur daily. Stress puts some of us constantly on edge. Some people live in a perpetual state of stress with periods of increased stress layered on top.

Good evidence supports the fact that people who are perpetually angry, hostile, and contemptuous have higher rates of heart disease, perhaps due to the chronic release of stress hormones.

To relieve stress, we often seek other outlets that are not good for our health. For example, after a really bad day, you might eat out of control or reach for a cigarette. Clearly, stress increases alcohol and drug use.

The Costs of Stress

Stress costs businesses money through higher health insurance premiums, more and longer disabilities, and inefficient workers. Stress costs families in tension and divorce. Stress causes more illness including heart disease.

In 2002, we bought nearly $17.2 billion worth of antidepressants and antianxiety drugs, an increase of nearly $3.7 billion since 2000.[72] Sales of stress management programs and products annually ring up more billions of dollars, offering stress-reducing services to individuals and corporations.

A study published in the *Journal of Occupational and Environmental Medicine* found that workers reporting depression and elevated stress levels posted 70% higher health care costs than those not affected by such conditions.[73]

How Not to Reduce Stress

While we may start out with the best of stress-reducing intentions, we bring our stressful lives into our quiet time. Too often, we create "quiet time" that is as hectic as the rest of our frazzled lives. We go on vacation, but we take our business cell phones or we check e-mail, so we never really get away. We spend time at the beach, but we get in line early to fight the crowd for the best beach chairs. We don't grocery shop and cook while we're on holiday, but eating out becomes a noisy, crowded, and expensive hassle. Somehow the idea of peace and quiet gets lost.

If you've retreated to the porch in the evening to get away, can you still hear the television? Or did you take your cell phone? Don't take your cell phone. The ringing will jangle your nerves, and the call will invade your peaceful moment. Ask yourself this question: "Do I have to answer the phone every time it rings?" Can't you let voicemail or the answering machine do its job? Then you can deal with the call later. Ask this question too: Is the call likely to be important? It could be your brother-in-law stuck in traffic. He just wants to while away the time as he sits amid the gridlock. Think of ways to protect the space you make for yourself.

Surveys and studies indicate that many people exercise to relax. I'm all in favor of exercise, but not competitive, high-stress exercise. Next time you go to the gym, look around. Observe the workout routines and ask yourself who is relaxing. Not the guy lifting weights and watching the televised football game (as a TV in another corner blares the news). Not the young woman diligently following a 90-minute workout she downloaded from the Internet onto her Palm Pilot—she is busily recording with precision her minutes on the StairMaster. Not that middle-aged woman promoting a business deal on her cell phone as she walks on a treadmill. Nor the guy sculpting his pecs to perfection, counting each weight repetition and watching himself in the mirror. This is relaxing? These people have simply converted work stress into fitness stress.

YOU NEED A PLAN

Just as with the other poor health habits discussed in this book, the impact of your daily stresses is cumulative. Moreover, your stressors run the gamut from big to small. I cannot tell you how to fix the big stressors in your life, like the boss who cuts the size of your territory every time you reach your sales goals. But if you reduce the effect of the other stressors in your life, you may be able to cope with your boss a little better.

So what should you do? Change some of your stressors and learn to change the way you respond to stress. These are the health choices that we all need to make. The important thing to know is that you do have choices. Here are some things to consider.

Stress comes in many forms and at different times in your day; therefore, you need a variety of methods to lower your stress. For example, you survive a tense meeting and need to release the stress. Depending on the meeting, sometimes you may need to exercise, while other times you may need to meditate to rid yourself of the stress. Sometimes stress relief requires music, sometimes silence. Sometimes it means being alone for a while, and other times it means talking with a good friend. You must find what works well for you when coping with different kinds of stressful situations.

Give yourself quiet time. You need to find a sense of serenity, of internal peace and quiet, of acceptance, of understanding. Does that sound almost impossible in the world you've grown used to? You can do it!

Did you notice the important thread common to the idea of time for yourself? Just being alone, *being you* for a while. No multitasking. No phone. No record keeping. Give yourself the gift of time and use it to put the stressful events into perspective. Then try to forget them for a while. This gift to yourself is a conscious attempt to steal a moment in which you can reflect, enjoy the quiet, and maybe give yourself a chance to daydream. Such moments help put the outside world in its proper perspective and help you regain your inner balance. These moments and times enable us to see the larger meaning to our lives.

Get away, even momentarily. Meditate, sit quietly in the park, hike in the mountains. Think of your own best quiet moments.

Try to do them more often. Do not let other disturbing thoughts enter your mind; if they do, invite them to leave.

Learn to meditate. Learn to center and calm your thoughts through either sitting or walking meditation. A simple but enormously effective calming exercise can be done by focusing all of your attention on the breath. Just breathe in and out through your nose calmly. Pay attention to how the breath feels, how your body moves as it breathes. Do not react or respond to the random thoughts that will come into your mind as you breathe. Return your attention to your breathing. Concentrate on your breath and the act of breathing. The phone call you have to make can wait another ten minutes. Three to 20 minutes, any amount of time will relieve stress.

Exercise. Exercise is a great stress reliever. But you need to exercise with the idea of listening to yourself as you exercise. Exercise may mean a long brisk walk along the bike path, or a slow walk through your neighborhood park.

Raise your awareness. Start by noticing the things that stress you—try to become more aware of the times when you are feeling stressed and why you feel that way. At the same time, try to observe when you feel peaceful, calm, or relaxed. Let me share with you a very revealing detail. When I give talks about stress, typically, two or three people approach me after the talk to tell me they *never* feel relaxed or calm. For some people, the process of de-stressing is a lot like stopping smoking. People have become addicted to the hypercaffeinated rush of stress. For some it is the necessity of shuttling between soccer and ballet lessons. Others are hooked on the feeling of importance by being able to work longer and harder than anyone else. Do you know any workaholics?

Just as you make a health choice when you decide whether to walk or to drive to the store, you need to make conscious choices about reducing the stress in your life. For example, think about how to answer these questions:

◆ If you want to get some exercise, why not try a quiet activity like yoga or stretching?

◆ When you want to sit quietly, can you still hear the television? Is anyone even watching it, or is it just on?

◆ Is the project you are working on so very important? Is there a way to simplify it or do it more efficiently? Must it be perfect, or does *perfect* often get in the way of *good enough*?

◆ Are you in the office longer than anyone else because you volunteered for the project? Or because you are just less efficient? Or is your life too cluttered to be efficient?

◆ Very few people on their deathbed say, "I wish I had spent more time at work."

The choice and method to lower your stress is less clear-cut than choosing to eat an apple instead of an ice cream sundae. The process is also less tangible. However, with practice, you can soon start to notice the difference—and your body will thank you for making the small changes. Managing stress is different for everyone. Some people will exercise. Some will walk. Others will paint and draw. Some will garden. Some will meditate. The only right answer for stress relief is the one that works for you.

When you find what works, you will soon feel calmer and less stressed. Along the path that leads you through your days, you'll start to find a few havens where there used to be none. By taking time out to counter stress, you can fortify and multiply these havens. In our modern world, you cannot have a stress-free life. But you can have a life in which stress does not lead you to bad health choices, a life where it is easier to play and work, a life where others find it easier to live with you. You'll also find it easier to live with yourself.

Chapter 10

WORK WITH YOUR PHYSICIAN

If you need major surgery or high-tech medical care, there's no better place to be than in an American hospital. Modern medicine can be truly miraculous when you are sick.

Your best medical goal, however, is to *prevent* disease in the first place. That's what this book has been about. As a physician, I look at treatment as a failure of prevention. By reading the chapters that preceded this one, you now know much more about prevention. You have the knowledge to make informed decisions to substantially reduce your risk of disease.

Even if you follow the first six recommended steps to maximize your own best health, there's still one more level of prevention you should use to your advantage: your physician. You can and should regard your physician as yet another way to keep you healthy and out of the hospital. Modern medicine can help you prevent a heart attack by identifying and lowering abnormal cholesterol values and blood pressure, and it can screen for premalignant conditions to reduce your risk of cancer.

By seeing your doctor regularly, you reduce your risk of heart disease, diabetes, and cancer as much as possible. The first six prescriptions for health contained in this book will keep you as healthy as possible, but you also have to remember that your past lifestyle and genetic heritage can put you at higher risk for certain conditions. Your doctor can help you combat these histories.

And one more thing: our parents and our grandparents trusted their doctors to keep their patients healthy—as though patient health lay in the doctor's hands. Not so. You must assume some responsibility for knowing about your own health and acting on that information, just as you take care of your own bank account.

THE MODERN VIEW OF HEART DISEASE

The ease with which modern medicine treats heart disease almost makes a heart attack seem too easily remedied. A heart attack? Take an aspirin, go to the emergency room, go through a procedure to dissolve the clot and open the blocked vessel, go home, return to your normal life. It's almost as if the heart attack never happened.

It's a fact that doctors have lots of answers for heart problems: bypass surgeries, angiograms, stents and pacemakers, and transplants, if necessary. However, while all of this technology can save a life, people don't think about the fact that these remedies cannot return the heart to a disease-free state.

While modern medicine can treat heart attacks effectively and efficiently, the truth is that once your arteries harden and become blocked, your life expectancy is shortened and your medical future is altered.

The real danger is that for a few hundred thousand people a year, their heart attack is the first, only, and last manifestation of their heart disease. Their heart attack is fatal.

There's also a second all-important point to consider. A heart attack is the end stage of a disease process that took decades to develop. This time gives you an opportunity for prevention.

A heart attack or stroke is the result of atherosclerosis or hardening of the arteries, a disease 30 or 40 years in the making. It is the end result of a process of chronic damage to the fragile inner lining of the artery by deposits of cholesterol, inflammatory cells, and other gunk (sorry for the big scientific word here).

Dr. Bob says:

◆ *The road to better health and a more vibrant and zestful life goes* around *the hospital, not through it.*

The Cost of Treating Heart Attacks

A tremendous amount of energy and money is spent treating heart disease. It is, after all, the number one killer in America. The Centers for Disease Control report:

◆ Heart disease kills more Americans than the next seven causes of death combined.

◆ 2,600 Americans die from heart disease every day.

◆ About 200,000 Americans under the age of 65 will die from heart disease this year.

◆ Ten times as many women will die of heart disease as die from breast cancer this year.

◆ The Steps to a Healthier US report from the Department of Health and Human Services estimates heart disease costs over $350 billion annually.[74]

◆ The direct costs for health care exceed $200 billion and lost productivity accounts for an additional $140 billion. One-quarter of the lost productivity amount is due to disability that results in unemployment, and three-quarters is due to premature death (death before age 65).

These numbers are huge. While we spend the money to fight the good fight, we more often spend the money *after* the heart attack has occurred. The truth is that we spend very little money to prevent the heart attack in the first place.

The goal of this book is to prevent that heart attack. Previous chapters have explained what the best science says and how to make lifestyle choices to reduce your risk of a heart attack as much as possible. At the start of the book, I quoted Dr. Claude Lenfant, who noted that we should be able to reduce heart disease 80% by changing our lifestyle. We have not yet met that goal. We have a long way to go.

Estimating Your Risk for a Heart Attack

Most people underestimate their risk of heart disease, an unfortunate and often fatal miscalculation—especially since doctors can identify and treat the risk factors and so prevent the heart attack.

Among heart disease patients, 80% have at least one of the major risk factors. The major risk factors include:

◆ family history of early heart disease

◆ smoking

◆ abnormal cholesterol and other blood lipids

◆ high blood pressure

◆ diabetes

◆ obesity

◆ physical inactivity

You can avoid heart disease by minimizing the known risk factors. People without such factors have only about 20% as much risk of heart attack as everyone else. Your goal is to develop habits that put you in the low-risk column in table 20.

Table 20			
RISK FACTORS FOR HEART DISEASE			
Factor	Minimal Likelihood	Moderate Likelihood	High Risk
Smoking	None	Past smoker	Current smoker
Total cholesterol	Under 200	200–240	Over 240
LDL cholesterol	Under 100	101–159	Over 160
HDL cholesterol	Over 60	40–60	Under 40
Blood pressure	Under 120/80	121–139 / 81–89	Over 140/90
Weight as BMI	19–25	26–29	Over 30 and especially over 35
Activity	Exercise daily	Some but inconsistent	Sedentary

CALCULATING YOUR HEART DISEASE RISK

Because most people substantially underestimate their risk for serious heart disease, you should know your cardiovascular-risk score—for the same reason you know your bank balance. Both measure where you stand. And once you know your score, you can do something about the numbers if you don't like them.

There are national calculators to help you determine your risk of heart disease. These short, simple, and very informative calculators are based on the excellent work of the Framingham Heart Study and the National Cholesterol Education Program. They ask about your age, your total and HDL cholesterol, your blood pressure, whether or not you smoke, and if you have high blood pressure. With this information, the calculator then gives you two pieces of information: it translates your risk of heart disease into a percentage and compares your score to others in your age group.

Look at the excellent one-page summaries that the National Cholesterol Education Program (NCEP) calculators developed. I strongly suggest you calculate your risk. Or go to the American Heart Association web site at americanheart.org to get more complete information on how to apply these numbers and assess your risk score.

Table 21

CALCULATE YOUR RISK OF HEART DISEASE
OVER THE NEXT TEN YEARS (MEN)

Source: National Heart, Lung, and Blood Institute, www.nhlbinih.gov/about/framingham/risksabs.htm

Find and Total the Corresponding Points for Each Factor

Age	Points
20–34	-9
35–39	-4
40–44	0
45–49	3
50–54	6
55–59	8
60–64	10
65–69	11
70–74	12
75–79	13

Total Cholesterol	Points at Ages 20–39	Points at Ages 40–49	Points at Ages 50–59	Points at Ages 60–69	Points at Ages 70–79
<160	0	0	0	0	0
160–199	4	3	2	1	0
200–239	7	5	3	1	0
240–279	9	6	4	2	1
≥280	11	8	5	3	1

	Points at Ages 20–39	Points at Ages 40–49	Points at Ages 50–59	Points at Ages 60–69	Points at Ages 70–79
Nonsmoker	0	0	0	0	0
Smoker	8	5	3	1	1

HDL	Points
≥60	-1
50–59	0
40–49	1
<40	2

Systolic BP	If Untreated	If Treated
<120	0	0
120–129	0	1
130–139	1	2
140–159	1	2
≥160	2	3

Your Risk of a Heart Attack in the Next 10 Years Based on Your Total Points

Point Total	10-Year Risk	Point Total	10-Year Risk
<0	<1%	9	5%
0	1%	10	6%
1	1%	11	8%
2	1%	12	10%
3	1%	13	12%
4	1%	14	16%
5	2%	15	20%
6	2%	16	25%
7	3%	≥17	≥30%
8	4%		

Table 22

Calculate your risk of heart disease over the next ten years (women)

Source: National Heart, Lung, and Blood Institute, www.nhlbinih.gov/about/framingham/risksabs.htm

Find and Total the Corresponding Points for Each Factor

Age	Points
20–34	-7
35–39	-3
40–44	0
45–49	3
50–54	6
55–59	8
60–64	10
65–69	12
70–74	14
75–79	16

Total Cholesterol	Points at Ages 20–39	Points at Ages 40–49	Points at Ages 50–59	Points at Ages 60–69	Points at Ages 70–79
<160	0	0	0	0	0
160–199	4	3	2	1	1
200–239	8	6	4	2	1
240–279	11	8	5	3	2
≥280	13	10	7	4	2

	Points at Ages 20–39	Points at Ages 40–49	Points at Ages 50–59	Points at Ages 60–69	Points at Ages 70–79
Nonsmoker	0	0	0	0	0
Smoker	9	7	4	2	1

HDL	Points
≥60	-1
50–59	0
40–49	1
<40	2

Systolic BP	If Untreated	If Treated
<120	0	0
120–129	1	3
130–139	2	4
140–159	3	5
≥160	4	6

Your Risk of a Heart Attack in the Next 10 Years Based on Your Total Points

Point Total	10-Year Risk	Point Total	10-Year Risk
<9	<1%	17	5%
9	1%	18	6%
10	1%	19	8%
11	1%	20	11%
12	1%	21	14%
13	2%	22	17%
14	2%	23	22%
15	3%	24	27%
16	4%	≥25	≥30%

These calculators interpret your overall risk and put it in perspective, giving you a clear understanding of your risk of heart disease. They also underscore the importance of smoking, cholesterol, and blood pressure. If your risk of heart disease is high, you should go to the doctor, who will treat these abnormalities and reduce your risk. If you do not know your cholesterol levels or your blood pressure, it's time to see your physician.

You'll notice that these calculators also highlight the importance of the lifestyle changes we have been reviewing in this book. As the research shows, most Americans do not follow a heart-healthy lifestyle. And even some of those who do faithfully follow the plan the book describes will still find they have abnormal cholesterol levels or blood pressure. This is where your physician can intervene and provide effective medications to prevent that heart attack.

TAKE YOUR MEDICINE!

You and your physician can reduce your risk of heart disease by identifying and treating your abnormal cholesterol values and your blood pressure. Even with the best of lifestyles, you still may need a prescription medication to optimally control your cholesterol and blood pressure. You can help manage your health by knowing your own numbers and by taking medicine, if necessary.

Unbelievably, abnormal blood pressure and cholesterol levels often go unmeasured or untreated. Even more frustrating for those of us in the prevention business, half of the people with high cholesterol or high blood pressure who are put on medication stop taking it within a year. The medications do not prevent heart disease if the little pills stay in the bottle.

Do you remember Marcie from chapter 5? Marcie did stop her exercise program once her neck and back pain lessened. Once again, she was too busy to be concerned with her own health. She returned to her daily routine of excessive work, stress, poor eating, and inactivity.

Marcie plowed through life too busy to take stock of her own heart health. She dutifully saw her gynecologist for mammograms and Pap smear testing, but she had not gone in for a complete physical for several years. Besides, everything used to check out so well. Finally, she went in for a compete physical only to find that she weighed much too much (no surprise there), her total cholesterol was very high, her HDL cholesterol was low, and her blood pressure needed treatment.

Her physician talked to her about the need for a heart-healthy diet. The doctor also told Marcie that she needed to exercise and control her weight. She nodded in agreement and then, of course, did little.

Six months later, she returned to the doctor only to discover that her cholesterol values and blood pressure were the same. At this point, her physician gave Marcie prescriptions to control both conditions. She was to return in three months for repeat blood testing.

Marcie took the medications faithfully for the three months. Her cholesterol levels improved wonderfully, and although her blood pressure required a second medication, it, too, was headed in the right direction.

Gradually over the next several months, Marcie began to forget to take her medications. She never totally forgot them, just some of the time. The pills did not make her feel any different, and she was busy. She didn't think missing a dose or two would hurt.

Of course, the question for Marcie is, will skipping medications make any difference?

Treating cholesterol or blood pressure is like prescribing eye glasses for reading. When you wear the glasses, you can read easily. When you don't, you can't. When you take cholesterol medications, your cholesterol drops toward normal. When you don't take your medicine, it goes back up.

Fortunately, there are several very effective medications to treat elevated cholesterol levels. Interestingly, one of these medications, the statin family, reduces heart disease more powerfully than predicted.

The problem occurs with people like Marcie who stop taking these highly effective, low-side-effect medications. These people stop taking the pills because they don't feel any different. You won't feel different; that's not the point of the medication. The medication works behind the scenes, so to speak. If you were given a prescription to lower your cholesterol, use the American Heart Association Risk Calculator, once with your before treatment numbers and then again using your after-treatment cholesterol numbers. (Doctors call these numbers *values*, as in valuable to know). The difference in numbers would show you your lowered risk of your heart disease. The medication is doing its job, even if you don't feel it. Remember this difference: your goal is to prevent your heart attack.

Keep Your Bad Cholesterol Low and Your Good Cholesterol High

Cholesterol is not just one simple blood fat. While there are multiple kinds of cholesterol and even sizes of cholesterol, the two basic cholesterols remain the most important targets. Your goal? Your total cholesterol, an easy measure marker for the bad LDL cholesterol, should be as low as possible, and your good HDL should be as high as possible.

The first thing you want to do is learn what your total and HDL cholesterol levels are. The next time your blood is tested, ask for a copy of the lab report. Do not accept a simple statement of "they are okay." Get the numbers. This is your life, and you need to have some control—and knowledge is the first step in taking control.

Then compare your numbers to the targets of the National Cholesterol Education Program panel. Table 23 shows a breakdown of the numbers.

Table 23	
TOTAL AND HDL CHOLESTEROL LEVELS SHOWING THE TARGET GOALS	
Total cholesterol	
Desirable	Under 200
Borderline high	200–239
High	Over 240
HDL (good) cholesterol	
Desirable	More than 60
Low	Under 40

WHAT DOES SCIENCE SAY?

The Multiple Risk Factor Intervention Trial (also known as MRFIT) studied 350,000 Americans and found a continuous graded relationship between total cholesterol and heart disease. *Graded* means that a person with a total cholesterol of 250 has a higher risk than a person with a cholesterol of 200, who has a higher risk than a person with a cholesterol of 175.

Keep in mind that HDL cholesterol is the good cholesterol, or think of "H" as "helpful" cholesterol. You want your HDL cholesterol to be as high as possible. An HDL level above 60 protects you. An HDL level below 40 for men and below 45 for women is associated with increased heart disease risk, almost regardless of your total cholesterol level.

One evening after a busy day and a frozen pizza for dinner, Marcie developed a little chest fullness, burped a few times, and slowed down. The fullness passed. Not worried and wanting to assure herself that there was nothing wrong, she went about her evening. The next day, Marcie's schedule was packed, and she tried to forget the fullness, although she had a nagging feeling in the back of her mind that this was more than a normal burp.

Two weeks later, while on the phone at work trying to deal with an unfriendly client, she developed that feeling of chest fullness, which quickly progressed to the point of pain. She felt sheepish and far too embarrassed to ask for help. Fortunately, her assistant came into the room just then, took one look at Marcie's ashen skin color, and called 911. Thirty minutes later, Marcie was in an excellent emergency room and diagnosed with a full-blown heart attack. Thirty minutes later, she was on her way to the cath lab for an angioplasty to open her blocked coronary artery. Doctors found the blood clot in her left coronary artery, dissolved it, and inserted a stent to keep the artery open. Thirty-six hours later, Marcie was given a lecture on a heart-healthy diet, given a total of four medications, and sent on her way.

Now the question becomes: Will Marcie be a slow learner or a quick study? Marcie needs to do a lot of changing to get her life and her health back in balance. One can only wonder—Marcie's behavior to date has not been promising.

KNOW YOUR BLOOD PRESSURE AND TREAT IT BACK TO NORMAL

Your blood pressure can be easily measured, but you should measure it only after a short rest since blood pressure rises with activity. Even though you will see some variability between readings, there is a general pattern. Hypertension, or high blood pressure, tends to increase with age. Currently, 30% of Americans have high blood pressure—that's 50–70 million adults with hypertension.

There is a consistent relationship between increased blood pressure and increased risk of heart disease and stroke. The majority of hypertension occurs with other cardiovascular risk factors, which further increases the risk. The blood pressure numbers associated with the lowest risk are a reading below 115/75.

Table 24

BLOOD PRESSURE CRITERIA OF THE JNC 7, JOINT NATIONAL COMMITTEE ON PREVENTION, DETECTION, EVALUATION, AND TREATMENT OF HIGH BLOOD PRESSURE

	Systolic (top number)	Diastolic (bottom number)
Normal	Under 120	Under 80
Pre-hypertension	120–139	80–89
Hypertension stage 1	140–159	90–99
Hypertension stage 2	More than 160	More than 100

As with cholesterol, when we talk about blood pressure, the best blood pressure is a low blood pressure. And as with cholesterol, lifestyle changes help the condition, but often only marginally so. Most patients with hypertension require treatment. The good news is that there are many good medications to lower your elevated blood pressure.

Look at these similarities between cholesterol and blood pressure:

◆ Half of the people who have high blood pressure do not know it—just as with cholesterol.

◆ Non-drug treatment, such as diet and exercise, is always helpful, but often it's only marginally effective at getting blood pressure back to a value that no longer requires treatment.

◆ Half of the people who are given medication to treat the condition do not take the medication regularly.

◆ If people don't take the medication, it does not work.

◆ For every 5 mm that your medication reduces the diastolic number, your risk of a stroke drops by 40%. Is that enough incentive to take your blood pressure meds?

Reduce Your Heart Attack Risk

Heart disease is largely preventable. People can and do get old without ever developing heart disease. A few of them are genetically lucky. Others follow a very healthy lifestyle—not just one part of a healthy lifestyle, but *all* of the health-promoting parts. These people also know their risks and take preventive medications when necessary.

I hope that by now you are better informed so you can substantially reduce your risk of heart disease by not smoking, exercising regularly, maintaining a normal weight, avoiding unhealthy food, and eating healthy food. Now add this to your to-do list. You should also have your cholesterol and blood pressure measured. You should calculate your risk of cardiovascular disease. And if necessary, you should treat your cholesterol and blood pressure levels to get them to normal. Only then will people with already high numbers see their risk for a future heart attack start to drop.

REDUCE YOUR RISK OF CANCER

Cancer is a difficult disease to treat unless it's found early. Fortunately, you and your physician can work together to prevent two of the three leading forms: lung cancer and colon cancer. Doing this would nearly halve the number of cancer deaths in this country. The first three causes of cancer death in women are lung, breast, and colon. The first three causes of cancer death in men are lung, prostate, and colon. Lung and colon cancer are unusual kinds of cancers because they are preventable.

AVOID LUNG CANCER. DO NOT SMOKE.

The best way to stamp out lung cancer is to stop it from ever starting. If all smokers stopped smoking today, the incidence of cancer of the lung, throat, and mouth would fall 90% in 10 years. Cancer of the bladder, kidney, and cervix would also fall. This is not trivial. The facts from the National Institutes of Health are astonishing:

◆ Lung cancer is the most common cause of cancer death for both men and women.

◆ Lung cancer accounts for 23% of all cancer deaths in women; 42% of all cancer deaths in men. The death rate is higher in men because they start smoking before women, and men also smoke cigars and pipes and chew tobacco.

◆ Compared to a nonsmoker, a man who smokes increases his risk of lung cancer by 2,000%, and a woman increases her risk by 1,200%.[75]

If you smoke or use tobacco, your physician can help you quit. This may be the best cancer-prevention treatment you can get from your physician.

SCREEN FOR COLON GROWTHS BEFORE THEY BECOME CANCER

Screening can make colon cancer a disease of the past. Screening finds colon polyps before they become malignant. This makes colon cancer unique among cancers. In all other cancers, doctors detect cancers only after cells have become malignant. With colon cancer, however, doctors have the opportunity to find small growths (polyps) in the colon *before* they start to turn malignant.

The accepted theory is that colon cancer grows in large colon polyps. A polyp is a little like a smooth wart, although the colon polyp grows more slowly. Both a wart and a polyp start as a small 1-mm smooth growth and slowly enlarge. The polyp grows about 1 mm in diameter a year. To put the size in perspective, compare the polyp to the "o" in this typeface. The "o" is about 2 mm. After 10 years, the polyp is 10 mm in diameter, or close to half an inch. Cancer typically develops in polyps that are 10 years old, or 10 mm in diameter. The purpose of colon cancer screening is to find the polyp while it's in the midsize range, before it becomes malignant.

If you haven't thought of screening for colon cancer—or you've avoided the idea because you think the colonoscopy test is uncomfortable or embarrassing—you are not alone. Talk to your doctor. Only 40% of adults have had any sort of colon cancer screening, so there is room for improvement.

Colon cancer runs in some families. If you have a family history of early colon cancer or if multiple family members have developed colon cancer, you are listening to alarm bells ring. The younger the age at which colon cancer appears (especially if the cancer was diagnosed before age 45 or even 50) and the more family members that are involved, the higher your risk. Discuss your family history with your physician. And be prepared to start screening when you are young.

SCREENING FOR OTHER CANCERS

As you might guess, I am in favor of talking with your physician about screening for other common cancers. Typically, the leading cancer screens include breast cancer for women, prostate cancer for men, and a skin exam for both men and women.

All cancer screening involves risk-to-benefit considerations. No test is perfect. As with any screening test, both false positives (positive results in the absence of real disease) and false negatives (negative results when the disease is really present) are possibilities. Each has its own costs. A false positive result may lead to an unnecessary surgical biopsy procedure. A false negative means the disease is present but was missed, a very different kind of risk.

At this time, the U.S. Preventive Services Task Force, USPSTF, recommends mammograms every one or two years for women over the age of 40. The USPSTF data shows that mammograms significantly reduce deaths from breast cancer. Unfortunately for men, there is no clear consensus on when to start screening for prostate cancer, in part because the test is too new, and in part because the studies have not been completed. This is an area for personal discussion with your physician. Your physician is your resource, just like your insurance agent, your financial adviser, and your accountant.

The point of this chapter is to tell you that while you can work at the other six lifestyle choices independently, this lifestyle choice is different. It requires collaboration and cooperation. Find a doctor you like and trust. Go in for physical exams. Follow the advice that he or she gives you, whether that is diet, exercise, taking medication, or undergoing screening procedures. Yes, you can do much to promote your health on your own. However, there are times you need professional help and prescription medication. The combination of making informed choices along with the contribution of modern medicine covers your health completely. Why would you do any less for yourself?

Chapter 11

CONCLUSION

LIFE IS NOT A SPECTATOR SPORT

Have you ever played a doubling game? Some parents use the game to teach children how small amounts of money can grow and accumulate. Here's how it works. Using a sheet of paper on which is printed a calendar with 30 boxes, one for each day of a month, the parent begins by writing 1¢ on the calendar's very first day. It doesn't seem like much, starting with a penny. The child is skeptical. On the next day's square, the parent writes 2¢, and on the third day, the parent writes 4¢, and so on.

By the end of the first week, the parent and child are recording 64¢ in the seventh calendar box, Saturday's box. To the child, this is an interesting exercise, but it doesn't seem to be going anywhere. It's been a week, and doubling has only accumulated pocket change, but to humor Mom and Dad, the child keeps going.

Suddenly things begin to get interesting. By the end of the second week, the total is $81.92. By the end of the third week, the total is an amazing $10,485.76, and by the fourth Saturday, with the help of a calculator, the parent and child are entering $1.3 million in the 28th box. Imagine where the numbers go from there with each passing day.

At the beginning of the game—or at the end of the first week, for that matter—if the parent had asked the child, "Which would you rather have, $1 million dollars right now or the total of doubling your money over 30 days?" most children would take the $1 million. They couldn't dream of a single penny adding up to $5.3 million in 30 days. They would have shortchanged themselves by $4.2 million. Incredible.

Table 25 A PENNY DOUBLES						
Sunday	Monday	Tuesday	Wednesday	Thursday	Friday	Saturday
$.01	$.02	$.04	$.08	$.16	$.32	$.64
$1.28	$2.56	$5.12	$10.24	$20.48	$40.96	$81.92
$163.84	$327.68	$655.36	$1,310.72	$2,621.44	$5,242.88	$10,485.76
$20,971.52	$41,943.04	$83,886.08	$167,772.16	$335,544.32	$671,088.64	$1,342,177.28
$2,684,354.56	$5,368,709.12					

Such is the power of slow and steady accumulation over time. Now apply this thinking to your health. Think about the days, months, years, and decades of inactivity, harmful food, lethal cigarettes, and other poor health practices. Every day, your body is assaulted with another wave of something that damages it from yet another direction: too much alcohol, too much stress, too much weight. While we may think of this as getting older, we're fooling ourselves with that excuse—almost giving ourselves permission to keep on living the way we have been.

Remember that chapter 3 explained that *aging is a process, not a disease.* Well, here we are: the first generation in the history of the world to have a chance to reach 85, 90, or maybe 100. We've got the opportunity to do this, unlike our parents or grandparents, who may have fallen far short of even age 75. But having the potential is one thing. Making it happen is quite another.

It won't just happen—not with our 21st-century lifestyle. If we keep battering our health with fast-food and stressful days...if we continue sitting in front of computer screens and televisions...if we remain content to watch other people play sports...we will not only throw away our longevity, we will saddle ourselves with unnecessary diseases and disability.

Yes, our days are busy, and we probably don't think too much about how we live. But somewhere, in the back of our mind, we think, "I really should lose weight, we really have to start eating better at home." "I really should get some exercise." "I really ought to quit smoking." But then the obstacles arise: With the kids' activities, we just never seem to have time. "I'll get serious about this as soon as the season is over, maybe when the kids are older... Maybe next month... After I get this project done... For sure, next summer...." In our day-to-day lives, we neglect the little voice in the back of our mind. It's easy to put off such thoughts, especially because we could honestly say that we didn't know where to start, even if we had the willingness to do so.

Well, that's changed.

If you've read this book, you know what to do. Not only are you a member of the first group in history to have the chance to live to 100, you now have a road map to help you get there. You know you can make informed decisions and choices about your own health. And now you know what healthy people know.

Here are Dr. Bob's seven prescriptions:

1. *Don't smoke.*

2. *Exercise for 30 minutes four or more days a week.*

3. *Maintain a Body Mass Index between 20 and 25.*

4. *Eat a diet high in colorful fruits, vegetables, whole grains, fish, nuts, and monounsaturated and polyunsaturated oils.*

5. *Drink small to moderate amounts of alcohol to help your heart.*

6. *Manage your stress.*

7. *See your doctor for preventive care and screenings.*

By following these seven lifestyle choices—keeping in mind the do's and don't's that scientific studies support—you can alter your life, invigorate your days, avoid preventable disease, and live longer. Should a soccer schedule or a project at work put off such vital goals? I don't think so.

Consider this your pep talk. You can use the principles of the doubling game to add vigor and extend your life with each new day on the calendar, or you can double your risk for heart attack, diabetes, or cancer. You have been informed; the choice is yours. How are you feeling these days? A little more sluggish, a little less limber? Do you huff and puff when you climb the stairs? Do you want to keep trudging down the same path, doubling as you go? Or do want to explore this new path?

The new path represents change, which is always hard. But, as the chapters tell you, you start with a few minor changes, and every day you change a little bit more for the better. You have to think beyond the first few days to appreciate long-term benefits. Focus on the momentum that you are starting to pick up. As you feel better, you'll want to do more. It will be a self-motivating experience: the better you feel, the better you'll want to feel.

So why bother to choose a healthier life?

You bother because good health does not just happen. You bother to make small everyday decisions because health choices, like the pennies, might seem insignificant at the beginning, but they add up. You continue to make healthy choices across the board—fewer bad foods, more healthy food, more exercise, managing your stress, and occasionally helping your heart by raising a glass to yourself to celebrate your new life. The idea is to start slowly and accumulate good health habits. These informed choices will enrich your life—you'll live longer and better, be more active, have less disease, and who knows? You might even break 100. You bother to choose because it does make a difference.

If you want more proof, ask the healthy people—they know.

EPILOGUE

Dr. Henry Blackburn, one of the original researchers in the Seven Countries Study, wrote a piece in 1970 describing the low risk male. His piece is reproduced with his permission below:

Let me sketch the "real low-coronary-risk male," who we have documented to live on the Isle of Crete:

He is a shepherd or small farmer, a beekeeper or fisherman, or a tender of olives or vines.

He walks to work daily and labors in the soft light of his Greek isle, midst the droning of crickets and the bray of distant donkeys, in the peace of his land.

At the end of his morning's work, he rests and socializes with cohorts at the local cafe under a grape trellis, celebrating the day with a cool glass of lemonade and a single, hand-rolled, hand-cured cigarette of long-leafed Macedonian tobacco.

He continues the siesta with a meal and nap at home, and returns refreshed to complete the day's work.

His midday, main meal is of eggplant, with large livery mushrooms, crisp vegetables and country bread dipped in the nectar that is golden Cretan olive oil.

Once a week there is a bit of lamb, naturally spiced from grazing in thyme-filled pastures.

Once a week there is chicken.

Twice a week there is fish fresh from the sea.

Other meals are hot dishes of legumes seasoned with meats and condiments.

The main dish is followed by a tangy salad, then by dates, Turkish sweets, nuts or succulent fresh fruits. A sharp local wine completes this varied and savory cuisine.

This living pattern, repeated six days a week, is climaxed by a happy Saturday evening. The ritual family dinner is followed by relaxing fellowship with peers. Festivity builds to a passionate midnight dance under the brilliant moon in the field circle where the grain of the region is winnowed.

Our Cretan, in the presence of admiring friends, is a man dignified in bearing, happy in countenance, and graceful in the dance.

On Sunday he strolls to worship with his children and wife. In church he listens to good sense preached by the Orthodox priest, a respected leader involved with his own family as well as his political and religious responsibilities.

Then our truly low-risk male returns home for a quiet Sunday afternoon, chatting with family in the shade, cooled by the salubrious sea breeze that is gently perfumed by smoke from olive-wood charcoal grills and fragrances of herbs and fresh animal dung wafted from nearby fields.

This man of Crete gazes peacefully on a severe but harmonious landscape. He is secure in his niche in a long history from the Minoans and before, a human in the long line of humanity.

He relishes the natural rhythmic cycles and contrasts of his culture: work and rest, solitude and socialization, seriousness and laughter, routine and revelry.

In his elder years, he sits in the slanting bronze light of the Greek sun, enveloped in a rich lavender aura from the Aegean sea and sky.

He is handsome, rugged, kindly—and virile.

His is the lowest heart-attack risk, the lowest death rate, and the greatest life expectancy in the Western world.

Finally, though healthy, he is prepared to die.

This, then, is a portrait of the man truly most free of coronary risk of all men on earth.

TABLES AND CHARTS

Tables

21. Calculate your risk of heart disease over the next ten years (men)

22. Calculate your risk of heart disease over the next ten years (women)

23. Total and HDL cholesterol levels showing the target goals

24. Blood pressure criteria of the JNC 7, Joint National Committee on Prevention, Detection, Evaluation, and Treatment of High Blood Pressure

25. A penny doubles

Charts

1. Average life expectancy from birth

2. Number of expected deaths per year by age for a healthy, average, and unhealthy group of 1,000 men

3. Number of expected deaths per year by age for a healthy, average, and unhealthy group of 1,000 women

4. Percent alive by age — smokers compared to nonsmokers

5. Percent of physically inactive people by age

6. Death rate over 12 years according to average distance walked per day

7. Death rates for men by quintiles of fitness

8. Death rates for women by quintiles of fitness

9. Relative risk of death by BMI

10. U-shaped curve describing how alcohol consumption affects longevity

Self-assessment tests

1. How much exercise do you get?

2. What color is your diet?

3. What's your stress level?

NOTES

[1] John W. Rowe and Robert L. Khan, *Successful Aging* (New York: Random House Inc., 1998).

[2] Meir J. Stampfer, Frank B. Hu, JoAnn E. Manson, Eric B. Rimm, Walter C. Willet, "Primary Prevention of Coronary Heart Disease in Women through Diet and Lifestyle," *New England Journal of Medicine* 343 (July 2000): 16–22.

[3] Anthony J. Vita, Richard B. Terry, Helen B. Hubert, James F. Fries, "Aging, Health Risks and Cumulative Disability," *New England Journal of Medicine* 338 (April 1998): 1035–1041.

[4] Elizabeth Somer, "Are kids eating too much sugar" WebMD (October 22, 1999).

[5] Susan Dominus, "Life in the Age of Old, Old Age," *New York Times* (Feb 2004): 26–58.

[6] Ibid.

[7] http://aoa.gov/prof/statistics/2001pop/factsforfeatures2001_pf.asp.

[8] Richard Singer, "The Application of Life Table Methodology to Risk Appraisal," in *Medical Selection of Life Risks* by R. D. C. Brackenridge and John Elder (Stockton Press, 1998).

[9] National Vital Statistics Reports Vol. 51, No. 5, March 14, 2003.

[10] Jess Mast, "Tobacco," in *Medical Selection of Life Risks* by R. D. C. Brackenridge and John Elder (Stockton Press, 1998).

[11] Edward Lew and Jerzy Gajewski, *Medical Risks, Trends in Mortality and Time Elapsed,* Chapter 3 (New York: Praeger Publishers, 1990), quoting studies based on L. Breslow and J. E. Enstrom, "Persistence of Health Habits and Their Relationship to Mortality: Preventive Medicine 9 (1980): 469–83.

[12] http://www.cia.gov/cia/publications/factbook/rankorder/2102rank.html.

[13] Public Policy Institute of California, http://www.ppic.org/main/pressrelease.asp.

[14] Press Trust of India, "Indian Immigrants live longest in California," Hindustan.com.

[15] American Cancer Society web site, Questions about Smoking, Tobacco, and Health. http://www.cancer.org/docroot/PED/content/PED_10_2x_Questions_About_ Smoking_Tobacco_and_Health.asp.

[16] Richard P. Sargent, Robert M. Shepard, Stanton A. Glantz, "Reduced Incidence of Admissions for Myocardial Infarction Associated with Public Smoking Ban: Before and After Study," *British Medical Journal* 328 (April 24, 2004):977–980.

[17] American Cancer Society web site on smoking, tobacco and health.

[18] lungusa.org/tobacco.

[19] Richard Doll, Richard Peto, Keith Wheatley, Richard Gray, Isabelle Sutherland, "Mortality in Relation to Smoking: 40 Years' Observations on Male British Doctors," *British Medical Journal* 309 (October 8 1994): 901–911.

[20] "Deliver Me from Temptation: The Danger of Just One Cigarette," Harvard Heart Letter, August 2002.

[21] James M. Lightwood and Stanton Glantz, "Short-term Economic and Health Benefits of Smoking Cessation: Myocardial Infarction and Stroke," *Circulation* 96 (August 19, 1997): 1089–1096.

[22] Ibid.

[23] JoAnn E. Manson, Frank B. Hu, Janet W. Rich-Edwards, et al., "A Prospective Study of Walking as Compared with Vigorous Exercise in the Prevention of Coronary Heart Disease in Women," *New England Journal of Medicine* 341(1999): 650–658.

[24] Ralph S. Paffenbarger, Robert T. Hyde, Alvin L. Wing, Charles H. Steinmetz, "A Natural History of Athletics and Cardiovascular Health," *Journal of the American Medical Association* 252 (July 27, 1984): 491–495.

[25] Min Lee, Chung-Cheng Hsieh, Ralph S. Paffenbarger Jr., "Exercise Intensity and Longevity in Men: The Harvard Alumni Health Study," *Journal of the American Medical Association* 273 (April 19, 1995): 1179–1184.

[26] Amy A. Hakim, Helen Petrovitch, et al., "Effects of Walking on Mortality Among Nonsmoking Retired Men," *New England Journal of Medicine* 338 (1998): 94–99.

[27] Urho M. Kajala, Jaakko Kaprio, Seppo Sarna, Markku Koskenvuo, "Relationship Between Leisure-Time Physical Activity and Mortality,"*Journal of the American Medical Association* 279 (1998): 440–444.

[28] Steven N. Blair, James B. Kampert, Harold W. Kohl III, Carolyn E. Barlow, et al., "Influences of Cardiorespiratory Fitness and Other Precursors on Cardiovascular Disease and All-Cause Mortality in Men and Women," *Journal of the American Medical Association* 276 (July 17, 1996): 205–210.

[29] Steven N. Blair, Harold W. Kohl III, Carolyn Barlow, et al., "Changes in Physical Fitness and All-Cause Mortality," *Journal of the American Medical Association* 273 (April 5, 1995): 1093–1098.

[30] Krucoff, Carol, "Keeping up with the young: the stiffness of aging may come from disuse—importance of exercise," *Saturday Evening Post* Nov-Dec, 1998 http://www.findarticles.com/p/articles/mi_m1189/is_n6_v270/ai_21279890.

[31] Miriam Nelson, *Strong Women Stay Young,* (New York: Bantam Books, 1998), p. 5.

[32] National Center for Chronic Disease Prevention and Health Promotion, Aug. 2003, http://cis.nci.nih.gov/fact/3_70.htm.

[33] David S. Feedman, Laura Kittle Khan, Mary K. Serdula, Deborah A. Galuska, William H. Dietz, "Trends and Correlates of Class 3 Obesity in the United States from 1990 Through 2000," *Journal of the American Medical Association* 288 (October 9, 2002): 1758–1761.

[34] Ali H. Mokdad, James S. Marks, Donna F. Stroup, Julie L. Gerberding, "Actual Causes of Death in the United States: 2000," *Journal of the American Medical Association* 291(March 10, 2003): 1238–1245.

[35] Nutrition Action Health Letter, March 2004, p. 3 (Dr Wansink's study).

[36] "Ice Cream Shops Serving Coronaries in Cones," Center for Science in the Public Interest, July 23, 2003.

[37] Sherry Baron and Robert Rinsky, Report of the National Institute for Occupational Safety and Health on mortality in football players, Jan 10, 1994, found at http://www.cdc.gov/niosh/hhe/reports/pdfs/1998-0085-letter.pdf.

[38] Gary Bray, "Health Hazards Associated with Obesity," Uptodate.com, written Jan 6, 2004, quoting Peeters, A, Barendregt, JJ, Willekens, F, et al. Obesity in adulthood and its consequences for life expectancy: a life-table analysis. *Annals of Internal Medicine* 2003; 138:24.

[39] Eugenia E Calle, Michael J. Thun, Jennifer M. Petrelli, Carmen Rodriquez, Clark W. Heath Jr., "Body-Mass Index and Mortality in a Prospective Cohort of U.S. Adults," *New England Journal of Medicine* 341 (Oct 7, 1999): 1097–1105.

[40] Gary Bray, "Health Hazards Associated with Obesity," Uptodate.com, written Jan 6, 2004, quoting Helmrich, SP, Ragland, DR, Leung, RW, Paffenbarger, RS Jr. Physical activity and reduced occurrence of non-insulin-dependent diabetes mellitus. *New England Journal of Medicine* (1991): 325:147.

[41] "New State Data Show Obesity and Diabetes Still On the Rise," December 31, 2002; http://www.cdc.gov/od/oc/media/pressrel/r021231.htm.

[42] JoAnn E. Manson, Walter C. Willet, Meir J. Stampfer, Graham A. Colditz, David J. Hunter, Susan E. Hankinson, Charles H. Hennekens, "Body Weight and Mortality among Women," *New England Journal of Medicine* 333 (Sept. 14, 1995): 677–685.

[43] National Cancer Institute web site, 3/16/2004. http://cis.nci.nih.gov/fact/3_70.htm.

[44] Amanda Spake, "America's Supersize Diet is Fattier and Sweeter and Deadlier," *US News and World Report* (August 9, 2002): 42.

[45] National Center for Chronic Disease Prevention and Health Promotion, "Preventing Obesity and Chronic Diseases Through Good Nutrition and Physical Activity" (August 2003), http://www.cdc.gov/nccdphp/pe_factsheets/pe_pa.htm.

[46] Gary Bray, "Health Hazards Associated with Obesity," Uptodate.com, written Jan 6, 2004, quoting, Narbro, K, Agren, G, Jonsson, E, et al. Pharmaceutical costs in obese individuals: comparison with a randomly selected population sample and long-term changes after conventional and surgical treatment: the SOS Intervention Study. *Archives of Internal Medicine* (2002): 162:2061.

[47] James Schoenberger, "Preventive Cardiology and Weight Loss," Uptodate.com, September 18, 2003, quoting SZ Yanovski, RP Bain, DF Williamson. Report of a National Institutes of Health—Centers for Disease Control and Prevention workshop on the feasibility of conducting a randomized clinical trial to estimate the long-term health effects of intentional weight loss in obese persons. *American Journal of Clinical Nutrition* (1999): 69:366.

[48] Ibid.

[49] Meir J. Stampfer, Frank B. Hu, JoAnn E. Manson, Eric B. Rimm, Walter C. Willet, "Primary Prevention of Coronary Heart Disease in Women through Diet and Lifestyle," *New England Journal of Medicine* 343 (July 2000): 16–22.

[50] Dr. Warren Thompson, Associate Professor of Preventive Medicine and Executive Health of the Mayo Clinic, 2002.

[51] Rob M. Van Dam, Eric B. Rimm, Walter C. Willett, Meir J. Stampfer, Frank B. Hu, "Dietary Patterns and Risk for Type 2 Diabetes Mellitus in US Men," *Annals of Internal Medicine* 136 (2002): 201–209.

[52] Michel de Lorgeril, Patricia Salen, Jean-Louis Martin, Isabelle Monjaud, Philippe Boucher, and Nicolle Mamelle, "Mediterranean Dietary Pattern in a Randomized Trial: Prolonged Survival and Possible Reduced Cancer Rate," *Archives of Internal Medicine,* 158 (June 1998): 1181–1187.

[53] National Institute of Cancer, "Obesity and Cancer, Questions and Answers," March 16, 2004, taken from http://cis.nci.nih.gov/fact/3_70.htm.

[54] K. McManus, L. Antinoro, F. Sacks, "A Randomized Controlled Trial of a Moderate-Fat, Low-Energy Diet Compared with a Low Fat, Low-Energy Diet for Weight Loss in Overweight Adults," *International Journal of Obesity* 25 (October 2001): 1503–1511.

[55] Walter C. Willett, *Eat, Drink, and Be Healthy,* (New York: Simon & Schuster Source, 2001), p. 17.

[56] Walter C. Willett and Meir J. Stampfer, "Rebuilding the Food Pyramid," *Scientific American* (Jan. 2003): 65–71.

[57] Kaumudi Joshipura, Frank B. Hu, JoAnn E. Manson, Meir J. Stampfer, Eric B. Rimm, Frank E. Speizer, Graham Colditz, et al., "The Effect of Fruit and Vegetable Intake on Risk of Coronary Heart Disease," *Annals of Internal Medicine* 134 (June 19, 2001): 1106–1114.

[58] Diane Hyson, *Health Benefits of Fruits and Vegetables: A Scientific Overview for Health Professionals,* p. 10.

[59] Harvard School of Public Health, Healthy Weight web site, http://www.hsph.harvard.edu/nutritionsource/healthy_weight.html#lessons.

[60] Key findings of the European Conference on Nutrition and Cancer, Lyon, France, June 2001, http://www.iarc.fr/EPIC/keyfind.html.

[61] Gundgaard, "Increased Intake of Fruit and Vegetables: Estimation of Impact on Terms of Life Expectancy and Health Care Costs," *Public Health Nutrition* (Feb. 2003): 6(1) 25–30.

[62] Harvard Heart Letter, October 2000.

[63] Jennifer Warner, "Whole-Grain Cereal Saves Lives, Choosing the Right Breakfast Cereal Could Make a Big Difference" Web MD, http://my.webmd.com/content/article/61/67445.htm?lastselectedguid={5FE84E90-BC77-4056-A91C-9531713CA348}, quoting *American Journal of Clinical Nutrition,* February 2003.

[64] Walter C. Willett and Meir J. Stampfer, "Rebuilding the Food Pyramid," *Scientific American* (Jan. 2003): 65–71.

[65] Walter C. Willet, *Eat, Drink, and Be Healthy: The Harvard Medical School Guide to Healthy Eating* (New York: Simon & Schuster Source, 2001), 73.

[66] Gary Fraser, "A Possible Protective Effect of Nut Consumption on Risk Coronary Heart Disease, the Adventist Healthy Study," *Archives of Internal Medicine,* 152: 1416–1424, July 1992.

[67] E.J. Feskens, D. Kromhout, "Epidemiologic Studies on Eskimos and Fish Intake," *Annals of the New York Academy of Sciences,* 683, 9–15.

[68] CNN Health Report, "Alcohol abuse up but fewer alcoholics," June 11, 2004, http://www.cnn.com/2004/HEALTH/06/11/alcohol.abuse.reut/index.html.

[69] Arthur Katsky, "Drink to Your Health," *Scientific American* (Feb. 2003): 75–81.

[70] Willett, *Eat, Drink, and Be Healthy,* p. 135.

[71] C. Hennekens, "Alcohol and Risk of Coronary Events." In: National Institute on Alcohol Abuse article, Alcohol and the Cardiovascular System. Washington, DC. US Department of Health and Human Services. 1996.

[72] Jeanne Sahadi, "The Cost of Stress," *Money Magazine* (March 21, 2003).

[73] Ron Z. Goetzel, David R. Anderson, R. William Whitmer, Ronald J. Ozminkowski, Rodney L. Dunn, Jeffrey Wasserman, and The Health Enhancement Research Organization (HERO) Research Committee, "The Relationship Between Modifiable Health Risks and Health Care Expenditures: An Analysis of the Multi-employer HERO Health Risk and Cost Database," *Journal of Occupational and Environmental Medicine* 40 (1998): 843–854.

[74] American Heart Association. *Heart and Stroke Statistics—2003 Update.* Dallas, TX: American Heart Association, 2002. Taken from http://www.healthierus.gov/steps/summit/prevportfolio/strategies/reducing/heart/burden.htm.

[75] Donald Shopland, "Cigarette Smoking as a Cause of Cancer," National Cancer Institute, SEER Data, http://rex.nci.nih.gov/NCI_Pub_Interface/raterisk/risks67.html.